'You wake up one day and realize the amazing impact these simple experiments have on your life'
Jacqueline

'*Wake Up!* is up there with the best things I've ever done, which means it's in great company with travelling to great cities, art galleries, getting married in Vegas, and climbing Ben Nevis and Snowdon with a short lung capacity'
Mark

'*Wake Up!* has given me fresh perspective and helped me find balance'
Vanessa

WAKE UP!

ESCAPING A LIFE ON AUTOPILOT

Chris Baréz-Brown

PENGUIN LIFE

AN IMPRINT OF

PENGUIN BOOKS

PENGUIN LIFE

UK | USA | Canada | Ireland | Australia

India | New Zealand | South Africa

Penguin Life is part of the Penguin Random House group of companies whose addresses can be found at global.penguinrandomhouse.com.

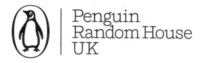
Penguin
Random House
UK

First published 2016

001

Copyright © Chris Baréz-Brown, 2016

The moral right of the author has been asserted

Designed by Hampton Associates, Aberdeen

Colour reproduction by Born Group

Printed in China

A CIP catalogue record for this book is available from the British Library

ISBN: 978–0–241–97742–2

www.greenpenguin.co.uk

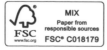

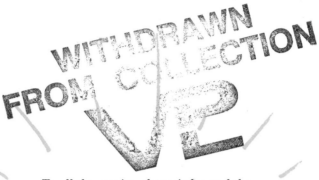

To all the crazies, the weirdos and the freaks. To all those who don't fit in but stand out. To everybody who knows that this is the most extraordinary of lives and it's happening right now.
To You: the awakening.

CONTENTS

INTRODUCTION

Over the years, I have noticed that I have not been myself.

I don't mean that somehow I have been out of sorts or physically unwell; I mean that someone else has been living my life. I have moments where I am deeply connected to myself, my family and friends, the work that I do and, indeed, this amazing planet on which we live. These moments are special. When they happen, I feel like I have absolute clarity. I am very present and very aware. There is absolutely nothing missing. In fact, everything is just perfect. When I experience those moments, I feel as if I truly connect to who I am and where I fit, in this wonderful thing called life. There are no fears, no worries and no concerns because everything is just right, and from this place I know that everything is fun, light and playful, and that the essence of this life is a fantastic game.

The downside is that this state is all too often fleeting, and before I know it I am back to leading a pinball life where I am bouncing around at ridiculous speeds, out of control and scoring points only by crashing into targets unintentionally. Then, by chance, I pop back out of it, a day, a week or even a month later, and I wonder what the hell's been happening.

Most of us have experienced driving from A to B and reaching our destination with no recollection of large chunks of the journey. We arrive safely and were in command of the vehicle throughout, and yet it feels as if somebody else was at the controls because we can hardly remember anything about getting there. We were driving on autopilot.

Truth is, this doesn't just happen while sitting at the wheel; this happens every day that we are alive. It happens at work, it happens at home, it happens in life, and this is what *Wake Up!* is here to address.

AUTOPILOT LIFE

The reason that most of our lives are spent on autopilot is due to the way our brains work. The brain works in two ways, consciously and subconsciously, and together this uses up a large chunk of our overall energy – around 25 per cent, according to many clever science folk.

The conscious brain is used for processes involving logic, rationality and higher levels of cognitive processing. When we are trying to decide whether leasing a car is better than buying one, or whether ground-source heat pumps will really make us a saving while helping the planet, we are using conscious processing. This takes a lot of energy, which is why when we tackle a particularly tricky intellectual challenge we often feel very tired quite quickly.

The subconscious brain, on the other hand, is a more efficient machine. It is adept at looking for patterns and similarities in what we are experiencing now compared to what we have experienced before. If something looks like a close enough fit to something from the past, the subconscious assumes they are the same and therefore directs our behaviour accordingly so that we respond in the same way we did last time. So, if we have noticed that the kitchen door no longer shuts as it should, when we are carrying two glasses of wine out and we don't the hear the tell-tale click of the latch, our heel automatically taps it in just the right place at just the right pressure to close it perfectly. Sweet. This takes no thought; and that is the beauty of autopilot.

It is a brilliantly efficient process that saves no end of effort and is absolutely necessary for us to function. We cannot consciously deal with every detail of our lives; if we had to do so, we would be exhausted. Just think how hard it is to learn a new language or an instrument, or even drive a car for the very first time. When we are carrying out menial tasks, things that are habitual or things that we have practised often enough for them to feel natural, then the subconscious is rather wonderful at conserving resources for use when we do things that are more taxing. The subconscious thinks faster and more 'automatically' than the conscious, which is why people who play tennis or the glockenspiel brilliantly have it to thank. They have practised to the point that the subconscious takes over and does a much better job than the slower conscious thinking. It's undoubtedly an exceptional performer in those situations, and it's important to make that distinction.

The challenge is that the subconscious has no 'off' switch. As we tend to live lives of habit with ingrained routines, most of what we do is stuff we've done before, and therefore autopilot becomes the default mode of existence. If we were a tennis player, that might be no bad thing, but most of us don't spend all our time on a tennis court – life is more complex than that. We therefore need to manufacture a better balance between the two systems of our brains. It is impossible to quantify what the right balance should be, or indeed the capacities of the conscious to run more of the show, but most of us know instinctively that if we can become a bit more awake and liberated from autopilot every day, it can make a huge difference to how we live our lives.

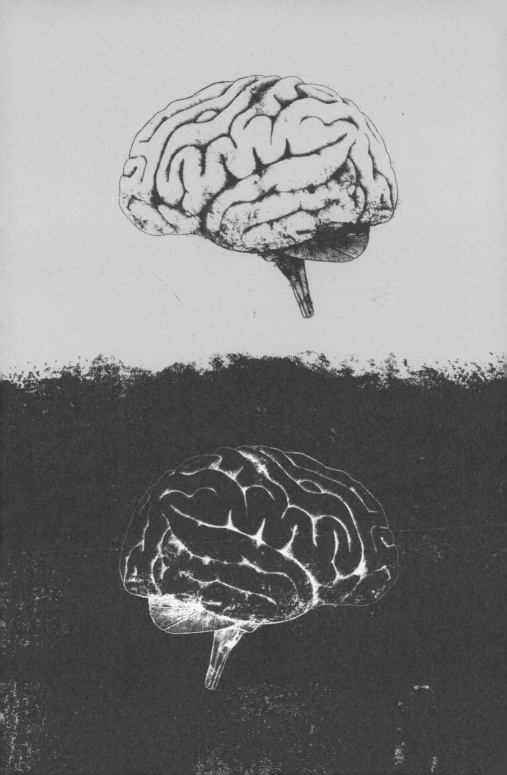

THE CAVEMAN BRAIN

The human brain hasn't evolved a great deal over the last 50,000 years, and we retain today survival instincts designed to protect us from prehistoric dangers, such as beasties wanting to eat us, rather than the perils of modern living.

To survive, we developed a mechanism within our brains that would spot potential dangers instantly and react to them immediately. It served us well back then, as the faster we reacted to even the vaguest of threats, the better chance we had of survival. Being fearful was therefore a key factor in your genes' procreation, so over time it became integral to humanity's DNA.

Those hazards are now long gone, and yet most of us still exhibit an instinctive aversion to risk. It's part of who we are.

When we are on autopilot we don't question that negativity bias, we just obey it. The caveman brain is hard wired to be wary of anything new and different, or anything that challenges our identity and what we know to have worked in the past. The caveman likes things to stay the same.

Of course, the caveman is only trying to help us. He is trying to keep us safe. He will never go away as he is part of our design. However, we can learn how to listen to him and respond rationally, rather than obey unthinkingly. When we notice him producing a fear response, pumping us full of adrenaline to encourage a fight-or-flight-or-freeze response, we can stop, breathe and ask what is really threatening about this situation? Often our inner caveman likes to stimulate a bigger reaction from us than is warranted.

While you are on autopilot the caveman is in charge; when you wake up he loses his grip.

Understanding how to listen to him, appreciate what he's telling you and then consciously choose what to do next is key to you finding liberation and leading a shinier life.

Let's consider the two halves of the conscious–subconscious spectrum.

SUBCONSCIOUS MIND

When we are on autopilot, our subconscious is in control. This means that we tend to be very reactive to the world in which we live.

When we experience any kind of emotion, we react, and our reactions dictate how our day goes. The subconscious loves fantasy and will entice us into a daydream whenever possible. Daydreams are usually about the past or the future and create a huge distraction from what is going on right now. When we are on autopilot we make snap decisions about everything, and very often they're bad ones. If we're feeling tired, we gulp down a sugary soda rather than taking a few minutes out to relax and recharge. If we've had a hard morning, the comfort of an overindulgent lunch might be what we reach for, making us inefficient for the rest of the day. It could be that the tasks we need to deliver today seem tough and pointless, so we turn to Facebook as a welcome distraction. Autopilot feels a little bit numb. It's passive. It's disconnected. When it kicks in we often feel as if we are very much on our own and that survival is our number-one priority. We lose awareness of who we are and what is important because we are driven more by instinct than by insight.

When we look in the mirror, what we see is what we believe we are, and nothing more: a name, a face, a fixed identity, with little connection to greater humanity. Time flies by, as in this state we are either busy with thoughts and fantasies and actions, or we enter a twilight zone in which our brains are drip fed by digital devices, social media, gaming, television, the morning newspaper . . . I call this the Shadowlands. When we are there, living on autopilot and always scared, because being scared means you are prepared for danger, we are living in a primal, almost animalistic way. Our subconscious may be efficient, but it ain't making us shiny.

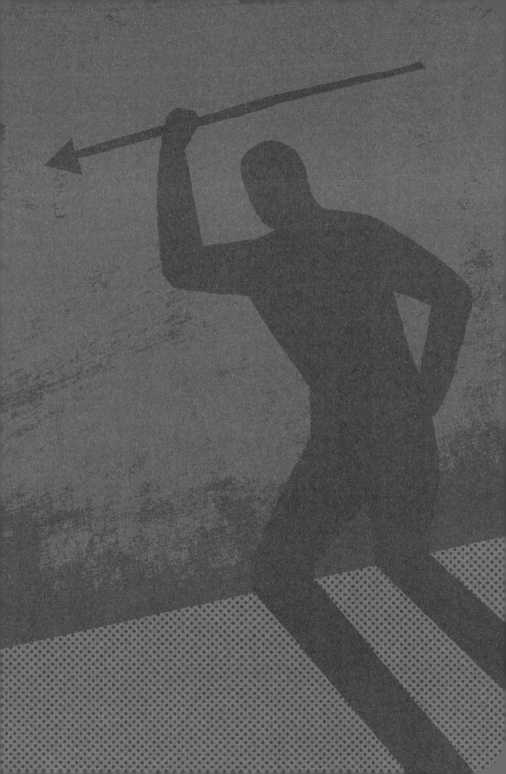

CONSCIOUS MIND

The opposite end of the spectrum is where we wake up. This is a truly connected and conscious state. We have all experienced such moments of crystal clarity. Fleeting glimpses of how wonderful life can be.

Often they are sparked by apparently random events: walking in the countryside on a particularly stunning day, or hearing a piece of music that literally strikes a chord with us. It may be as we hold a loved one close. Sometimes, and rather bizarrely, we feel more alive when death or disaster intervenes. The day before I wrote this, David Bowie died. Although it was a particularly sad day, there was something rather magical about it. I found myself more awake because of it, as I was reminded not only that, like Bowie, you can absolutely be who you want to be in this life and celebrate that fact every day, but also that nothing lasts for ever. A very useful perspective in staying conscious.

Everyone has their own experience of waking up to life. It's a common part of living. When we do tune in, we notice that we no longer react to the world around us but we respond more deliberately and with greater purpose. We seem to have a wider choice and can flex our perspectives to appreciate any situation from a positive point of view. Our mind quietens; we find it present and focused as opposed to its more erratic behaviour on autopilot.

When we wake up, we notice that we are anything but on our own; we are truly connected to everything and everybody on this planet because, energetically, we are all one. This heightened sensitivity helps us understand what is important and what is not and enables us to leave our petty obsessions behind so that we can focus on what really counts.

When we wake up, we become aware, we create, we harmonize with the world around us instead of trying to fight it and we find that everything becomes easier. For me it's a truly vital state of being (in both senses) and couldn't be more different from being on autopilot.

BREAKING FREE FROM AUTOPILOT

Autopilot is like sitting passively in front of your TV, constantly snacking when you're not even hungry and letting whatever is on the screen wash over you.

When you wake up, it feels as if you are starring in an award-winning TV programme you've created yourself, and that you will continue to do so every day you walk this planet. Just take this moment to ponder some of the times when you have felt fully awake and connected. Close your eyes, take a deep breath and remind yourself how it felt. Specifically, concentrate on what made the experience so enjoyable.

WHAT WAS YOUR MIND LIKE IN THAT MOMENT?

WHAT EMOTIONS BUBBLED UP FOR YOU AT THAT TIME?

WHAT WAS THE SENSE OF CONNECTION LIKE TO YOURSELF, TO OTHERS AND TO THE PLANET?

WHAT WAS IT ABOUT THIS MOMENT THAT FELT DIFFERENT FROM HOW YOU FEEL WHEN YOU ARE ON AUTOPILOT?

DRAW IT, WRITE IT, SCRIBBLE IT, CAPTURE IT HERE

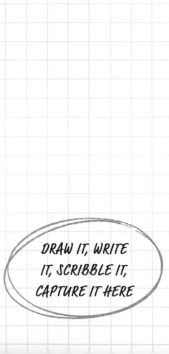

DRAW IT, WRITE IT, SCRIBBLE IT, CAPTURE IT HERE

One of my ongoing frustrations is that, although I have accessed this amazing state of wakefulness many times, it disappears all too quickly and I return to the treadmill of autopilot time and again. Ironically, that frustration helps encourage autopilot to take over more easily. When we try too hard we can take things far too seriously. To wake up we have to have fun and relax. It doesn't work from an uptight place.

The reality is that our subconscious is extremely efficient at taking over our minds, and will do so if given the slightest opportunity. Regardless of what blissful states we have encountered, as soon as we start to get busy and do things we have done before, autopilot will kick in to save energy. It's part of our design. However, I do believe that deliberately waking ourselves up more often can have a profound impact on the quality of our lives, the decisions we make and our general joie de vivre. The more frequently we do so, the more attuned we will be to that state and the weaker autopilot's grip will grow. It can never fully let go as we need it to survive, but it can become less dominant and therefore support us rather than rule our lives.

USING THIS BOOK

Before diving in and experimenting with the techniques this book offers to help you wake up, it would be a useful exercise to spend a day or even a week just noticing how often you feel truly awake.

Carry this book with you and jot down on the previous page whenever you notice it and what you think is responsible for it. When I tried this, I was stunned by how infrequently I woke up while working. I recently asked a group of people to audit themselves for a week, and each person came back surprised by how much of their life was dictated by autopilot. A couple of honest folk even said that during the test they couldn't think of one time they popped out of this soporific, habitual state, and then wondered just how much of their life had drifted by in the same way.

Rather sneakily, autopilot not only feeds off our existing habits, but also creates new ones. The caveman brain loves the familiar. Obviously, it thinks, something we have experienced and survived in the binary world of 50,000 years ago can't be that bad, so when we are on autopilot we will naturally choose options that we have chosen before. This results in large chunks of our lives becoming habitual and smothering us like a huge and downy comfort blanket.

I am a fan of meditation, mindfulness, yoga and many of the more esoteric schools, and have huge respect for these philosophies; however, I find that they are much better at getting me to work on my inner game than on my outer one. They help me manage my energy, attain focus and quieten my mind but not necessarily connect with the great big soup of this planet, humanity and universal consciousness. Personally, I need stuff to do as well as stuff not to do; it's the yin and yang of wake-up.

This book is designed to supplement such calming approaches with more gigglesome, action-packed and experimental play. I believe that the only way to wake up is deliberately to bring in new and different experiences to our lives that will provoke a heightened sense of consciousness as we engage with them. We are all unique, and each have different needs, beliefs, desires and identities, so different experiences will impact us in different ways and what works for one person might not work for another. Essentially, *Wake Up!* is a series of experiments for you to try out, play with and see which work for you.

Many of these experiments have been trialled among large groups of people and we know they have real potential for positive impact. Others are presented here for the first time, so you have the chance to be part of an even larger experiment. Tell us how they make you feel!

Above all, please remember that what you now have in your hands is an opportunity, not a burden. This is not a book that will add things to your to-do list to make even more demands on your time. Rather, these are just ideas for you to play with if it feels right. If you skip some, don't feel guilty. If some of them don't work for you, that's only to be expected – there's no way they could all be suited to one individual. There is no right or wrong way to do them and no correct order to do them in; just trust that, somewhere among them, you'll find what you need.

Some people benefit more by repeating an experiment on consecutive days; for example you might try something from Monday through to Thursday, then on Friday review and see what you've learned. There are spaces in the book for you to jot down your insights and learnings and outtakes as you go. Alternatively, some of you will find that doing an exercise just once is enough to get what it is about, and that is cool too. You might want to read the book from front to back and engage in everything in between, or just dip in and out when you need a little boost.

My only advice would be, don't just pick up this book, read it, and put it back on the shelf: you need to experience these experiments to shift your consciousness. *Wake Up!* is about less thinking and more doing. My good friend Jeremy once said to me, 'Chris, there are those who do and those who don't.' Be a doer and life will be forever richer. We cannot wake up intellectually, it has to be a holistic and energetic experience which can be provoked only through doing some fun stuff. Don't take it too seriously; it should be a giggle. I have deliberately gone light on research and statistics and all the clever-boffin embroidery, because that's not what this book is about. There is no real science of consciousness; just opinion, and this is mine. To quote from my last book,

'What counts can often not be counted, and what is counted often doesn't count,' and that's where I am coming from, for sure.

If you need more of a boost, do these experiments with a friend as their learning could well enhance yours. I've noticed that instantaneous enlightenment from them is rare; what more often happens is that small changes of awareness have an impact far greater than imagined. If you tune in to yourself as you try them out you are likely to notice some extraordinary results.

The movie *Lawrence of Arabia* is based on the life of T. E. Lawrence, a man who doesn't feel like he fits in and follows his own personal quest to find himself. In the desert, he makes a very unlikely connection with Arabian desert tribes. One of the most famous lines before the start of a challenging battle is, 'Big things have small beginnings.' While we are not all about to confront the Turks with our own band of armed Bedouin, we are each, in our own unique ways, making small changes that can potentially have a big effect on our lives if we allow them to.

If one of the exercises isn't quite working for you, feel free to adapt and bend and recreate it into something that does. The principles within them can be delivered in many ways, so make it fit for you. The exercises will help you either tune in and focus on something important (these are denoted by a head icon), plug in to one or more of the resources that are all around you (these are denoted by a lightbulb icon) or power up your body and/or your mind (these are denoted by a lightning-bolt icon). Each exercise is divided into three sections: an insight into the experiment, a plan to put it into action and the payoff you'll receive when you do.

My last top tip before letting you loose on all the fun is that the way you approach these exercises will dictate how much you get from them. If you go in half-hearted you will get half-baked returns. If you rush them they will certainly whizz you by! If you go in with an open heart and positivity, you will get abundance back. And before doing any of them, just take three deep breaths either sitting or standing straight, with a big smile on your face, and know full well that the adventure is about to begin. Strap yourself in.

IN SUMMARY

- Spend some time noticing how often you get off autopilot and wake up. What made it happen?
- See these experiments as a bit of fun that can only add sparkle to your life. It's not a job, it's a giggle.
- Before doing any of them take a moment to breathe deeply and put a smile on your face and you will get much more back.
- Feel free to adapt them so that they work for you, but just make sure you fully engage in them to get the benefit.
- Breathe.

I DON'T KNOW WHERE
WE'RE GOING FROM HERE,
**BUT I PROMISE IT
WON'T BE BORING.**

DAVID BOWIE

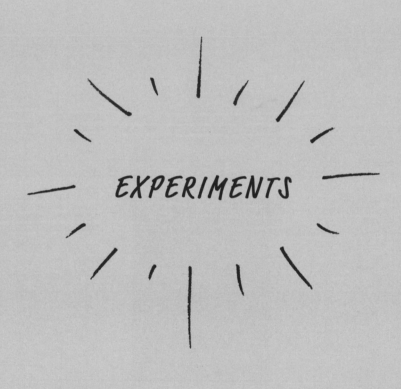

EXPERIMENTS

BREATHING

We each take about 20,000 breaths a day. The average human respiratory rate is thirty to sixty breaths per minute at birth, decreasing to twelve to twenty breaths per minute as adults. As babies, we all take deep, relaxing breaths from our abdomen. If you've ever watched a small child sleeping, you'll have seen their bellies rise and fall.

As we get older, the way we breathe changes. Especially when we are stressed or alarmed, our bodies operate on our more primitive 'fight, flight, or freeze' instincts and we take short, fast breaths to prepare for danger. Prolonged periods of stress mean we constantly breathe like this, only ever using the top third of our lungs. It's the bottom third of our lungs, however, that supplies two-thirds of our breathing capacity. So shallow, thoracic breaths mean we aren't getting what we need to function at our optimum level. As a result, our cognitive abilities go slack, we have trouble staying alert and connecting with others, and we often just have less fun.

On the flip side, when we breathe deeply we're likelier to have more energy and feel less stressed. Our posture and digestion can even improve. Breathing helps release toxins and strengthens our immune system.

Breathing properly is the fastest way to get off autopilot as it slows down the brain and gives greater clarity.

LEARN TO
Breathe!

THE INSIGHT

Generally, we are all useless at breathing. I learned how bad I was at it when I had to be coached for six months to learn how to do it properly.

When we breathe incorrectly, we starve our bodies of oxygen and therefore find it hard to achieve clarity and balance between our subconscious and conscious brains. When our brains are going too fast and don't have that balance we are naturally on autopilot. If we can just slow them down and get them to harmonize more, our sense of connection increases exponentially. I tend to find that most of my clients struggle to breathe deeply enough and therefore often find themselves reacting instinctively to the world rather than responding deliberately to it.

Without good breathing it is impossible to connect either to yourself or the planet, and all the fascinating and Technicolor energies therein.

THE PLAN

We are going to train your breathing so that when you feel that you have lost consciousness and you are living on autopilot, you can bring it back quickly and effectively just by nailing the breath.

I want you to spend three minutes breathing well, five times a day: when you wake in the morning, mid-morning, just after lunch, at around 4 p.m. and, finally, before you hang out with your loved ones.

Here's how that looks:

- Find a place where you feel comfortable that has little distraction and sit with your feet on the ground with a straight back and start by smiling.

- Then breathe in through your nose for five seconds and hold it for another six seconds.

- Finally, breathe out through your mouth for the final seven seconds.

- Repeat two more times or until you feel conscious and present and connected (stop if you get lightheaded).

So all you have to remember is 5-6-7, 5 seconds in, 6 seconds held and 7 seconds out.

THE PAYOFF

If there is one thing that you can do anywhere, at any time, which has the most profound impact upon how awake and connected you are, it's breathing.

Taking a few good breaths beforehand will enhance every exercise in this book. Poor breathing equals disconnect, which will let autopilot take over. By breathing well you will have a much clearer perspective, much greater choice and a chance to be bigger in your life.

Make breathing well a part of your everyday life and you can't help but wake up.

Kill

YOUR
TELEVISION

THE INSIGHT

When we are tired and feeling in the need of some comfort, the appeal of snuggling up in front of the television can be too good to deny.

All we have to do is press buttons to bring the world's best entertainment into our lives. It takes no effort and therefore we can truly switch off and let our over-stretched conscious brains shut down as our subconscious rolls around in the colourful wonderworld of the pixilation in front of us.

A little TV is not a bad thing, but a lot of TV is a waste of life. In the UK we watch an average of a little under four hours of TV a day; in America it's a little under five. For most of us our only time at home with our families is after work and it would appear that we are wasting too many of those precious moments with our loved ones by entering a televisual coma.

Not only that, television influences our worldview, increases the level of our dissatisfaction, manipulates our spending, and even decreases the regularity of our lovemaking. Naughty TV.

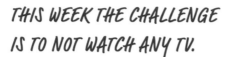

THE PLAN

THIS WEEK THE CHALLENGE IS TO NOT WATCH ANY TV.

Notice that when TV is not an option you have so many other things you could do that are truly rewarding. When you get home from work or finish your day's tasks, do something you wouldn't usually do instead of absent-mindedly vegetating in front of the box.

Read a book, go for a walk, phone a friend, learn an instrument, try some new recipes, hang out with your family and have a proper conversation about what life is like, meditate, grow something, sort out the attic . . . who cares what you do as long as it's a conscious choice and not in default autopilot mode.

A friend of mine, Ben Edmonds, decided that instead of watching TV he would learn some new skills, one of which was to make a knife by hand. As a result, he now owns Blok Knives, who make some of the best chefs' knives in the world and have a 3½-year waiting list for their exquisite goodies. What could you achieve if you didn't watch so much telly?

THE PAYOFF

The first benefit of not watching TV is that you will get a lot of time back; time you can use to enrich your life rather than just survive it. Over a week, if you usually watch the UK average amount; you'll get back a whole day of free time. That's a three-day weekend every week!

The second payoff is that by deliberately avoiding the passive state induced by television you will find that you will be more conscious and therefore more awake for more of your day, and so will find it easier to make better decisions, connecting with who you really are and those loved ones in your life.

Let's lead extraordinary lives and not just watch other people's.

INSTEAD OF TV,
THIS WEEK I THINK
I'LL TRY MY HAND AT...

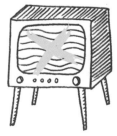

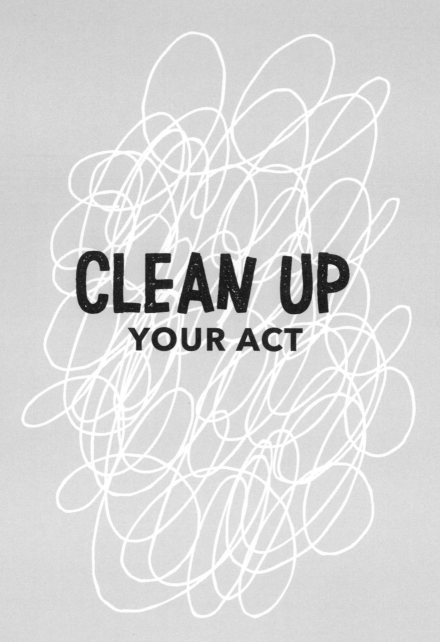

CLEAN UP

YOUR ACT

INSIGHT

When we are living our lives on autopilot our awareness suffers. We are not particularly aware of what our priorities are, the impacts we're having on the world around us and how we're looking after ourselves.

I am constantly struck by our ignorance as to what we put into our bodies just to get through the day-to-day challenges that we face. In any busy city you can see hordes of people who are largely sustained and stimulated by high doses of caffeine, refined sugar and alcohol.

When you are reliant upon these drugs it is very difficult to be fully conscious and aware as these little beasties are controlling your system and not you. They all work in their own unique way, but each one of these stimulants is amazingly effective at unbalancing you. Interestingly, we are probably more aware of the powerful impact that alcohol has and yet are often oblivious to the crack cocaine of the food industry, refined sugar. Recent research in France showed that laboratory rats chose sugar over cocaine – despite the fact they were addicted to cocaine.

THE PLAN

I am not suggesting that we should ban these stimulants for ever but I do believe that if we take notice of our bodies we'll be amazed at how we are poisoning them on a daily basis. So this week we're going to clean up our act.

FOR THE NEXT FOUR DAYS, BAN CAFFEINE, REFINED SUGAR AND BOOZE FROM YOUR SYSTEM.

It's as simple as that. So that means no lattes, no sticky doughnuts, no sweets, no sneaky drinks after work, no biscuits, no mass-produced gunk, no fizzy drinks, no glass of Barolo with dinner. The caffeine and the booze are relatively easy to spot but to avoid the refined sugar you have to look very carefully at the labels of what you eat – and, trust me, it's in nearly everything in ridiculously high doses.

Due to the highly addictive nature of these stimulants, especially the sugar, you may feel headachy and a little shaky without them. Drink plenty of water and eat small, frequent meals to help balance you out. The cold turkey will be short lived, so persevere, the payoff is huge.

THE PAYOFF

Just the process of thinking about how you eliminate them from your diet is a useful one. By doing so you will become more aware of how reliant we can become upon our little habits.

Many people, myself included, find that a simple detox has a profound impact. I personally find not having my Americano in the morning more painful than I ever imagined for the first couple of days, then its spell is broken and I can choose whether it is something that I want in my life or not, rather than acting only through addiction. When we consciously choose what we put into our system, we have already started to wake up and will reap the benefits energetically every time we turn down one of those naughty little hits.

This expansive way of looking at life, the universe and everything
CAN HELP US GAIN CLARITY AND REALIZE THAT
we are players on a small stage in a vast cosmic arena.

TRAVEL INTO SPACE

INSIGHT

Astronauts commonly experience a deep spiritual shift when they see the earth from space. They often realize that so much of their identity is based upon who they are on our planet and therefore the way they live their lives and what is important to them. Yet once they are physically separated from earth and are spinning around the 'blue dot' once every hour and a half, they find all their beliefs are challenged in the most liberating of ways.

Astronaut Chris Hadfield hit the press recently with his Space Oddity video, which went viral with millions of views. He says that when you are in space, 'you recognize the unanimity of our existence. The commonality.' He felt his video was so popular because 'It helped show people something I understand very well: that this is an extension of human consciousness. Human understanding. Human perspective on ourselves. We need to understand it and make it part of our increased self-awareness. This was a little step towards that.'

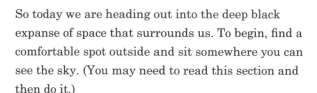

THE PLAN

So today we are heading out into the deep black expanse of space that surrounds us. To begin, find a comfortable spot outside and sit somewhere you can see the sky. (You may need to read this section and then do it.)

Taking a deep breath, smile and sit straight and then close your eyes and imagine yourself sitting in a space rocket.

Imagine the jets firing up and as the noise and vibration increase, feel yourself lifting up from this planet and see the ground beneath you getting further and further away as you accelerate into space.

Enjoy the ride.

Once you feel like you are approaching the moon, land there gently. Look back at planet earth and appreciate it for what it is.

It's your home and a place where mankind has achieved some incredible things. As you watch, notice how beautiful it is and how quiet it seems from space. There is a stillness that's quite intoxicating.

Soak it all in and notice any shifts that happen in you from this expansive perspective. Don't rush; it's not every day you can hang on the moon.

When you feel ready you can start heading home and, as you do so, enjoy your re-entry into the atmosphere, first seeing continents, then individual countries, expanses of water, mountain ranges, until eventually it's fields, cities, forests and roads.

Then land yourself comfortably back on the ground.

THE PAYOFF

The galaxy's greatest writer, Douglas Adams, summed it up well: 'The fact that we live at the bottom of a deep gravity well, on the surface of a gas covered planet going around a nuclear fireball 90 million miles away and think this to be normal is obviously some indication of how skewed our perspective tends to be.' This expansive way of looking at life, the universe and everything can help us gain clarity and realize that we are players on a small stage in a vast cosmic arena, and thereby reconnect with what is really important, not what shouts the loudest.

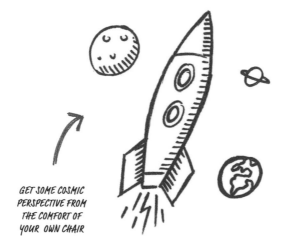

GET SOME COSMIC PERSPECTIVE FROM THE COMFORT OF YOUR OWN CHAIR

TUNE IN

We live fast-paced lives that are all about doing stuff. We are amazingly good at filling our days with activities and running from one thing to the next. When we are frenetic and focused on getting stuff done, it's very difficult to tune in to who we are and the world in which we live.

Much of this book is about helping us step back from that busyness and energetically reconnect with who we are and the world in which we live, so that we have a clearer perspective of why today can be extraordinary.

After years of being desensitized to the world we need to recalibrate our systems if we are going to make *Wake Up!* part of our everyday lives. The fastest and simplest way to start to reconnect with this sensitivity is to slow down. Sit or stand with a straight back, taking a huge breath deep into your belly, hold it a few seconds and then exhale, letting all the stress and complexity of life out with it (see page 28).

You know you have tuned in when

- you are aware of who you are, where you are and are present in the moment

- time slows down a little

- you are clear and focused

- you feel good, positive emotion

- everything feels right.

What you will find is that every time you tune in, it will become easier to do so next time. To begin with, you may have to be quite conscious about deliberately taking action to reconnect but over time you'll find yourself doing it quite naturally as it becomes ingrained in your neural and energetic pathways. With more practice, you will find that this heightened state of awareness improves in quality and clarity, and is sustained for longer.

Initially, when you start, that wonderful sense of awareness may only last a few seconds, but soon you'll find you will hold it for minutes and then, you lucky ones, hours. Some of you might be able to hold it consistently for days, weeks, or months or even years. I've never yet managed to get beyond a few hours, but many claim that, when they have made such profound connection, they never lose it, so let's hope that could be true for us all.

Before connecting to the energies outside of us, tuning in helps us get our energies ready.

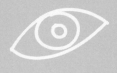

NOTICE
what you
NOTICE

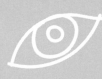
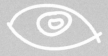
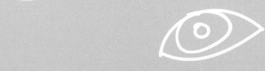
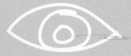

THE INSIGHT

Many years ago, I was working on a creative project in London. As part of an idea session I decided that a new perspective was required, and so my fellow creative and I decided to cross London Bridge imagining we were looking through the eyes of a child. It was a fascinating process. It took over an hour and a half and we had at least thirty ideas in that time, all stimulated by what we saw around us.

The project was designed to help our client avoid staff burnout by improving their management techniques. When we looked at the River Thames in all of its turbulence, eddies and tidal flows we noticed that the water was moving at very different speeds depending on which section we looked at. It struck us that our client only worked at one speed, which was flat out. The idea that came from the river was that each project would be designated as fast, medium or slow. They would be planned and scheduled according to their pace and each team member would be assigned a mix of each so that they could manage their energy better and have more time to reflect.

I would usually cross that bridge by foot in a matter of minutes and not see any of the world around me. To be awake to the world we live in we need to see more. Therefore, we're going to be doing some tuning in.

TUNE IN

THE PLAN

Everywhere you go for the next four days carry with you a small notebook and a pen.

WHENEVER YOU NOTICE SOMETHING THAT FEELS LIKE IT COULD BE INTERESTING TO YOU, NOTE IT DOWN IN YOUR BOOK.

These things could be people, conversations, buildings, articles, or a fleeting glance from someone in a passing bus. It doesn't matter what you find interesting; it only matters that you notice it.

For me the things that stand out tend to create some type of emotional reaction in me. If the emotion is noticeable then it is worth investigating why, as there may be something for me to learn. For you it may be something different. You may be far better attuned to sights than sounds, in which case, tune in to what you hear as you live your life and then notice which sounds and rhythms attract your attention. It may be that your life is too serious right now and that the things that grab you are those that are more playful and fun. Just notice what you notice.

THE PAYOFF

By deliberately noting down the things we notice we will become more sensitized to the world in which we live and therefore enjoy a heightened sense of connectedness and vitality.

Others who have tried this often report that they feel more attuned to the energy of where they are and start to experience more synchronicity. The more we notice, the more awake we become.

DRAW IT, WRITE IT, SCRIBBLE IT, CAPTURE IT HERE

COOK FROM
SCRATCH

INSIGHT

My relationship with food has developed markedly over time. I used to believe that the sole purpose of food was to put energy into my system so that I could live my life. Now I know better, beer and curry are no longer my best friends (although occasional buddies, for sure).

When you start to become more sensitive to energy, you notice very quickly that what you put into your body is what you get out. When we live our lives too fast, we can lose touch with that. When living on autopilot we are reactive to our needs. If we're feeling sluggish in the morning, we know some caffeine will perk us up. Mid-afternoon energy dip? Any snack laced with refined sugar will sort that out. Usually, we ingest this junk without even realizing we're doing it. Autopilot refuels us and doesn't care if it's the right fuel in the long run. It just cares about keeping us going now.

THE PLAN

BOTH AT WORK AND AT HOME, EAT ONLY FOOD THAT YOU HAVE PREPARED YOURSELF FROM RAW INGREDIENTS.

This means no prepacked snacks, no takeaways, and no processed rubbish. Source the freshest local ingredients that you can and you will notice the benefits. Visit your local greengrocer, butcher or fishmonger and enjoy the process of finding what's best today. Certain things will look riper and more glorious than others; pick them up, smell them and notice what attracts you. You may not have ever cooked before but don't worry because the internet has all the recipes for any dish you can imagine. Any shopkeeper worth their salt will direct you to the things that are in season and will always have their favourite way of cooking them. Ask them and you never know what you will learn. To make this work will require some planning and preparation; but it is well worth it.

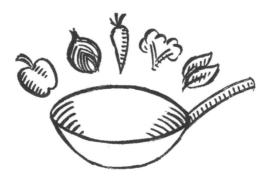

THE PAYOFF

After connecting more deeply with what we eat we will make better decisions about nutrition for ever. You will notice that certain foods give you much better payback than others. Through experimentation I have found that mass-produced bread is of no benefit to me, and therefore have cut it out of my diet. Without it, I have much better energy and am more consistent throughout the day. We are all different, of course, but by trying things out you will tune in to what suits you.

You'll also start to make friends with local shopkeepers and, by doing so, you'll know where your food comes from and become much more invested in it. The difference between mass-produced products and a lovingly created fresh dish is extreme; once you realize the benefits of eating fresh and how easy it is to deliver, it's hard to go back.

As Boy George once said, 'Never eat anything that has an advert.'

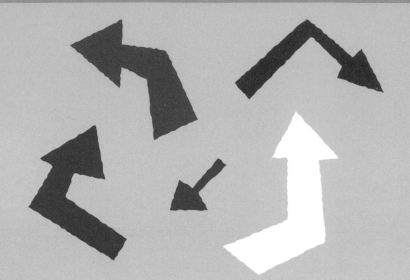

GET LOST
AT LUNCHTIME

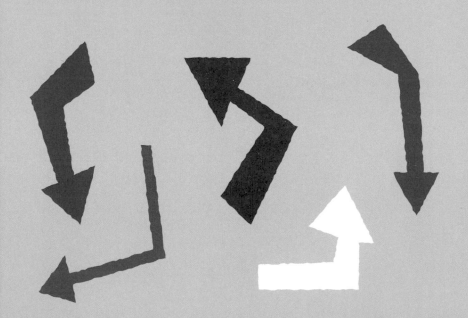

THE INSIGHT

Most of us are in almost total control of our own lives. We manage our time, money and environment so that there are very few opportunities to be surprised.

The computing power in our phones far exceeds the most advanced computers of twenty years ago and allows us to check our bank balances, train times, weather conditions, house thermostats, grocery deliveries and how many calories we burned today without doing any exercise at all. With GPS hidden in all our devices we never experience the exhilarating feeling of not knowing where we are, where we are going or how we might get back whence we came. Being lost and alone helps us with self-reliance and teaches us how to cope with the uncertain and the new in our lives. As author and adventurer Jon Evans explains, 'Eliminating "being lost" may sound good on paper, but strikes me as akin to settling into a very comfortable wheelchair without learning how to run.'

THE PLAN

THIS LUNCHTIME I WOULD LIKE YOU TO GO FOR A WALK AND GET LOST.

(If you are familiar with your immediate surroundings, just jump on the first bus or train you see that's heading for somewhere you've never been.) When I do this, I purely follow whatever attracts me and then I just see where I end up. You'll never be entirely lost as you can always ask for directions, but losing your sense of place is all part of the adventure; so enjoy wandering aimlessly.

As you wander, slow yourself down and start to pick up more of the details of the world around you. When walking in familiar places autopilot takes over. When walking somewhere new and different we will start to spot more intricate details of the world around us. The architecture, street names, the people living and working there, the smells and the sounds will all be slightly more tantalizing and may hold a few surprises. Much of this would not be noticed while walking on autopilot or looking down at your phone.

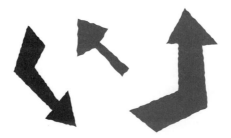

THE PAYOFF

When we are lost we tend to be in a more heightened state of sensitivity as we start to look for clues to find our way home. This sensitivity helps us become more awake and appreciate the environment in which we live. Getting lost also means by definition that we are drinking in new, rich and often surprising experiences, which helps us enjoy being alive that bit more.

PLUG IN

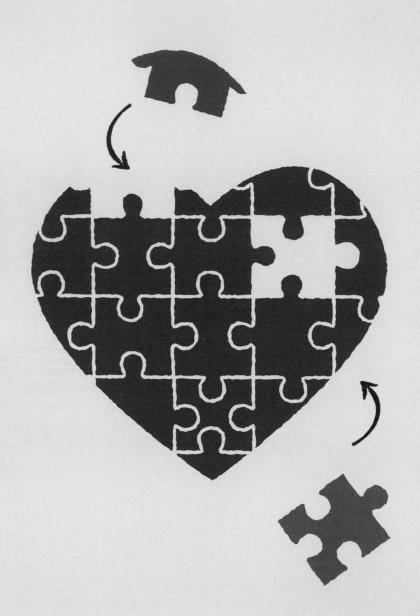

When you
CONNECT
*to what truly makes you
tick you will find you
will be more conscious*
**OF LIVING IT
RIGHT.**

Walkie

TALKIE

THE INSIGHT

The pressure and complexity of modern living often make it hard for us to find clarity. Our busy brains can be quite distracted just dealing with the stimulus of everyday living, so it's often a challenge to get down and dirty with what really counts in our lives.

A recent Harvard University study showed that, at any given time, an average of 50 per cent of the population is not focused on what they are doing. This was not the case twenty years ago, simply because the tools of interruption were not so plentiful.

We tend to construct narratives about who we are and what is happening in our lives, and often they aren't true. Common fallacies include lamentations about how we came to be in the situation we are in and why we have no way out. Something along the lines of, 'I can't follow my passion until the children have grown up; until then I must be a beast of burden.' We become wedded to these falsehoods as they seem to give us perspective when actually what they do is imprison us in a world of fantasy.

THE PLAN

To get past these stories and to help you connect
with the truth, take a little excursion with a friend.
Go for a short walk with him or her and while you're
walking, speak really quickly about your life: what's
working now and what's not, what's making you
happy or sad – just blurt out whatever comes into
your head. If you talk quickly enough, eventually
you'll run out of logical, clever or even truthful
things to say; at that point just say whatever comes
into your head and keep speaking quickly. As you
continue to talk, every now and again you will say
something that creates some type of state change in
you: those are the things of interest.

Your friend's role is just to listen to what you're
saying and maybe note down a few of what appear
to be the key points in your blurt. After ten minutes
of doing this, it's good just to land where you've got
to. You may notice that you've clarified an aspect of
your life that needed some attention. The greater
insight you've gained will, perhaps with a little bit
of thought over a cup of tea, help you decide how to
address it. Often after playing with this approach
people find that they know exactly what to do next.
The key thing is to write down what you are going to
do immediately; as the clarity in this rather beautiful
state can soon be lost when the busyness returns.

And, as good friends do, it would be nice to offer your
buddy a chance to do the same.

THE PAYOFF

If you do walkie talkie whenever you are stuck, you will find that you will become far clearer on how you live your life and far more conscious of how to make sure that every day is extraordinary. It is like pruning shrubbery – you need to clear out the old wood to encourage new growth. Once you put the work in to make the changes, everything will blossom. It's hard to be awake when you are living a made-up version of your life, but when you connect to what truly makes you tick you will find you will be more conscious of living it right.

MAKE A
PLANE
AND THEN FREE IT

THE INSIGHT

I used to know a guy who had a rather strange obsession. He used to love taking a Frisbee onto the top of a mountain and seeing how far it would fly. Although it turned out to be an expensive hobby as many were lost to the wilds, he loved the sensation of seeing them disappear into the distance.

We often live our lives feeling quite constrained and boxed in. It can feel as if the weight of the world is upon us and that pressure just squeezes us until we fit the mould.

Being frivolous and playful can easily be lost from our nature, and yet it is so much a part of our essence. Every day contains one thousand, four hundred and forty minutes, yet we only spend six of them laughing. Let's stash some more fun minutes in the daily time-bank.

THE PLAN

IT'S A SIMPLE ONE. MAKE A PAPER AEROPLANE, SAFELY GO SOMEWHERE REALLY HIGH AND SEE HOW FAR IT FLIES.

Watch where it lands so that it can be recovered, but most importantly enjoy its release and watch as the wind takes it on a journey.

Depending on the aerodynamics of your craft and the wind conditions of the day, it could go on the most marvellous adventures. Although we cannot see turbulence and wind currents, your plane will be living with them. A paper plane released upon high is not too dissimilar to the way our lives roll out. Their course cannot be predicted from the start, as there will always be some surprises. Some elements of life crash and burn superfast and some take the most wonderful circuitous routes to get to a place we could never imagine.

If there is something that's been bugging you, write it inside your plane before releasing it into the skies and, as you do so, literally let it go.

(Don't make the end too pointy if people are about; save the dart design for remote locations.)

THE PAYOFF

Just doing something for the pure joy of it can help us remember that this experience of being on the planet is most importantly about having fun. If we're not enjoying ourselves and loving the experience of being alive then we are truly wasting the glorious life we have been given.

There is nothing deep or clever or profound about paper aeroplanes but the smile on people's faces as they release them into the air is more worthwhile than any number of weighty and serious therapeutic processes. Be a kid again and let them fly.

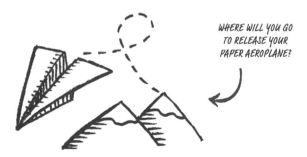

WHERE WILL YOU GO
TO RELEASE YOUR
PAPER AEROPLANE?

MAKE A PAPER AEROPLANE

1.

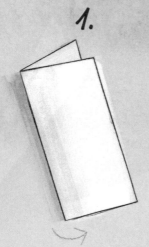

FOLD PAPER IN HALF (LONG-WAYS),
THEN FOLD BACK FLAT

2.

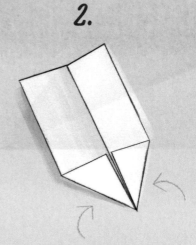

FOLD IN TWO CORNERS
TO THE CREASE

5.

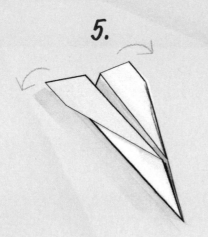

6.

WHAT ARE YOU WAITING FOR?!...

...FLY!

3.

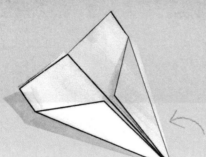

FOLD BENT CORNERS
TO THE CREASE AGAIN

4.

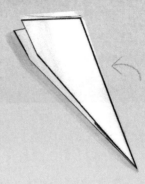

FOLD IN HALF

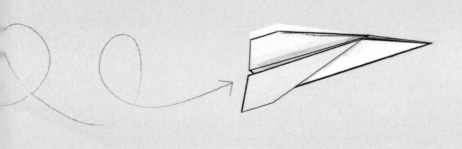

Spielzeug

INSIGHT

My good friend Dan Kieran introduced me to the concept of Spielzeug. His next book will be devoted to the concept, one so beautiful that I felt compelled to include it here. It is a German word, and simply means 'plaything', but, as is often the case, its essence is lost in translation.

Spielzeug relates to the palpable energy that certain objects have. Many of our favourite items have it; a pen, a coffee mug, a pair of glasses or, in my case, a guitar. Those things become our favourites because there is an energy within them that is different from the rest; an energy that personally connects with us. I believe this energy is not just within objects but also exists in buildings, art, places and people.

Some of you will be very aware of Spielzeug, others will not; but what is true is that if we attune ourselves to feel it more often, then every day we have a much greater chance to connect with our environment.

Connecting energetically to things around us will help us become more conscious of ourselves, and the world in which we live. It will therefore help us wake up and feel more alive.

THE PLAN

THIS WEEK SPEND TEN MINUTES A DAY QUIETLY HOLDING SOME OF YOUR FAVOURITE THINGS IN YOUR HANDS.

Taking one thing at a time, close your eyes, take a deep breath and notice how it feels. First, focus on feeling its shape, weight and texture, and then, letting go of that focus, simply hold it and allow yourself to connect more deeply.

If you have a favourite book, for example, once you have held it, pick up one that you have no connection with and contrast the difference.

You will start to notice how Spielzeug can live in the strangest places and in the most everyday objects. Certain buildings and locations will create a positive mental or physical sensation, while others will almost repel you. When you find somewhere overflowing with Spielzeug, sit there quietly taking a deep breath and smile as you enjoy what the energy gives you.

You will notice that certain people have this energy too. Some folk naturally create an energetic connection to you, making them somebody you want to be around. As the American author and poet Charles Bukowski said, 'The free soul is rare, but you know when you see it – basically because you feel good, very good, when you are near or with them.'

THE PAYOFF

Being able to feel Spielzeug is like having your own compass for living. By attuning yourself to it and using it to help yourself make decisions you will find that you start making better choices that fit you better energetically.

When you notice Spielzeug you will naturally feel more alive and more aware of who you are and the world around you. It's implicit in noticing, as to feel it, you have to be connected, and when you are connected you are awake.

Spielzeug is all around us. Tune in to it and make yourself feel more alive.

POWER UP

When we are tired, overstretched, depleted
and just plain pooped we don't have
the energy to balance out our thinking.
The conscious brain needs lots of juice and
without it the subconscious just takes over.

For us to wake up we need a good clean energy
system. The whole book is about energy; but the
distinction here is less to do with universal energy and
more to do with our personal energy. Our bodies and
minds need to be well looked after if they are to spark
in the right way. Without the right spark it is impossible
to wake up regularly and to hold that consciousness.

To Power Up we need to play some tunes physically;
through nutrition, exercise, sleep and rest. We also
need to learn how to get our minds working more
productively by dealing with negativity and fear,
getting more focus and being more open to possibility.
And then just as importantly we can get enormous
amounts of energy by encouraging more positive
emotions and becoming more playful, more excited,
and more sensitized to the world in which we live and
the way that we respond to it.

Elements of this book will focus on how you can get your energy to work better for you and how to make sure you have enough of it. We all have different engines and each needs to be tuned and balanced in its own unique way. Experts can help us understand how to do that, but the key to success is knowing when it feels right and when it feels wrong. When you tune in to that, you can spend the rest of your time experimenting to find out what it is that helps you resonate a positive, dynamic and livened energy.

You know when you get your energy right because you feel:

- vital and dynamic

- positive and optimistic and happy

- full of life

- balanced and open

- focused and clear.

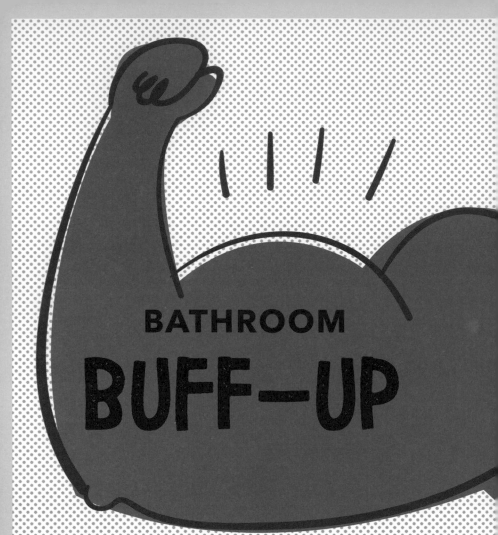
BATHROOM
BUFF–UP

THE INSIGHT

Before the invention of the alarm clock, Native Americans used their bladders to wake up at the right time. If they wanted to get up early they would drink plenty of water; if they wanted to get up later they drank only a little. It is a simple idea, but highly effective, and they used the method well into the twentieth century.

Recently I met a man who used a similar awareness to help him make sure he had energy throughout the day and stayed fit. Every time nature called he would do twenty press-ups. He explained that it gave him two great benefits. First, by exercising regularly throughout his day he found he had more energy at work and therefore was always at the top of his game. Secondly, he never had to invest the time to visit a gym and yet he was totally ripped.

The average modern Briton now spends more than twenty hours a day sitting or lying down. A recent study from the Department of Health states that only 6 per cent of men and 4 per cent of women manage the NHS recommendation of taking thirty minutes of moderate exercise five days a week.

THE PLAN

TAKE ADVANTAGE OF NATURE'S OWN ALARM CLOCK BY DOING SOMETHING PHYSICAL EVERY TIME YOU NEED TO GO TO THE LOO.

You don't have to do twenty press-ups; you could pull a plank for sixty seconds, do some sit-ups or burpees or strike a yoga pose. Choose whatever suits your body, your style and the space and facilities you have available.

The key thing is to do an exercise that gives you energy, and if you make it a habit you will see the benefits it gives you. By the way, you don't have to do the exercise in or indeed anywhere near the bathroom! After each visit, just find a space that feels good for you and do a one-minute workout. This takes a certain amount of courage if your only available space is an open-plan office, but you'd be amazed how envious your colleagues will be when you drop and give it twenty as if it's the only right and proper thing to do.

THE PAYOFF

By structuring in this simple and swift bit of physical exercise you will find that your energy will be more consistent through the day and that you will feel more awake.

Over a day this can make a huge difference to how alive you feel and to the positivity that you bring to the party. After just four days of doing this, you will already start to reap the benefits of being more buff. Buff brings confidence and general good vibes, which is key in keeping us out of the Shadowlands of autopilot.

Draw Life

AND GET
THE PICTURE

THE INSIGHT

It's all too easy to lose touch with what's going on for us and what is most important. As we get older it feels as if time accelerates as we assume more and more responsibility, and we can feel quite out of control of our lives.

The more things we do, the less time we spend on each activity, which means it becomes more of a struggle to engage properly with any of them. Micro-tasking is pretty unrewarding as everything feels as if it's only just about done and we never get to celebrate it, because as soon as it is finished we dive into the next micro-task. We can become whirling dervishes with no real appreciation of what's important and little appreciation of the fun. I have used this exercise for many years when connecting with my team, or even more recently with my son when we were having problems understanding each other.

THE PLAN

THIS WEEK I WANT YOU TO GRAB A FRIEND, FOUR BIG PIECES OF PAPER AND SOME COLOURED PENS.

Take ten minutes to draw what's been happening in your life over the last year. There is no right or wrong with this. Whatever comes into your head is just perfect, so get it down on the paper. You don't have to be a great artist as any squiggles can capture the essence of your experience, and I often find symbols and stick men go a long way.

Now shift attention to capturing on another piece of paper how you would like the next year to be.

Again take your time, have some fun and dream a little.

Ask your friend to do the same, again with no pressure or competition. Just enjoy.

Now comes the important bit. Take your time to explain your picture of the past and then your picture of the future to your friend and then listen to them explaining theirs. Soak it up and enjoy the connection as you listen to each other generously and get more insight into what's going on for each other.

THE PAYOFF

This simple approach tends to cut through a lot of the noise and fantasy stories (see Walkie Talkie, page 64) that we clog up our lives with and helps us land on the areas that have more emotional resonance.

There is no guarantee you'll have a breakthrough, but chances are if you play with this approach a few times with a few different people, you will start to get much greater clarity as to where you are and where you want to go.

For me the most interesting elements are not about achievements, material possessions or the houses in which we live, but more importantly it's the quality of living that shouts out from this exercise. Most of us draw how we want to be, rather than what we want to have. By nailing those elements, you will find that you will be more conscious of who you want to be every day and be driven to live that more, helping you be true to the unique and special soul that is your essence and waking you up to who you are.

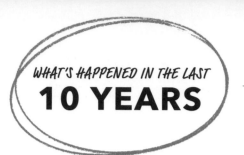
WHAT'S HAPPENED IN THE LAST
10 YEARS

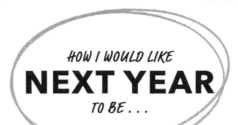

HOW I WOULD LIKE
NEXT YEAR
TO BE . . .

PLUG IN

It's very easy for us to live our days on this planet thinking that we are on our own. We believe that our lives are just ours to lead and that the struggles and hardship we suffer are only ours to bear.

Spiritual practices can help us deal with external factors by calming and balancing our inner energies, so that we are better equipped to deal with the life we lead. Once we have learned to calm our minds and increase our energy flows, we can connect more readily with the world around us.

Making this connection can take decades. I believe, however, that there is a shortcut to waking up if we plug in to the energies that we have around us every day and help them change our level of consciousness. For sure, we need to be tuned in to make that happen, but that is just one part of waking up. When we plug in as well, we take things to a higher level altogether.

Imagine that your body is a sports car and your mind its engine. We could spend years tinkering under the bonnet, tuning the engine to such a degree that it should theoretically outperform any of its rivals, but that serves little point if it never goes out on the track.

Far better to make some small adjustments, then take it out for a few laps and see how it performs, coming back with more information that will enable us to tune it to the next level.

Personally, I much prefer time on the track to time in the garage. Energy sources are all around us and some live in surprising places. You may find that you can plug in to places, times, people, sounds, perspectives, art, literature, food, the sea, animals, family, plants, yourself. By working out what plug-ins you have available, you will find that wherever you go you have a way of waking up just by flicking the switch.

My most powerful ones are being in, on or near the sea, properly connecting with people on what matters, being in nature, being in a busy city but stepping back and soaking it up. The list goes on.

You know that something is plugging you in when

- it helps you tune in

- it expands your perception beyond you and your usual awareness

- it gives you a positive energetic kick

- you feel connected to something much bigger

- everything becomes possible and nothing is a problem.

The wider our repertoire, the more we can vary it to what's needed here. And then we can wake up whenever we feel like it.

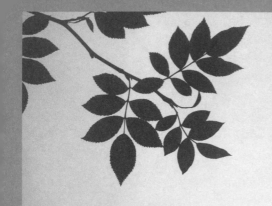

FIRST
TEN MINUTES

OUTSIDE

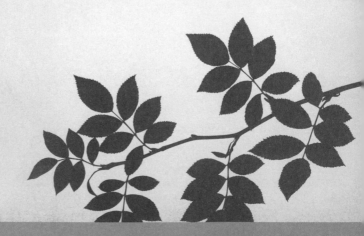

THE INSIGHT

Our days are getting packed ever more full with increased demands on our attention and efforts. We now consume about 100,000 words each day from various media, which is a massive 350 per cent increase over what we handled back in 1980.

Many of us feel as if time is escaping us because of the speed at which we lead our lives and the pace our constantly innovating society sets. Days blur into weeks and weeks into months. The Roman philosopher Seneca may have put it best two thousand years ago: 'To be everywhere is to be nowhere.'

When we start our day, we know we have a lot to do. The temptation is to leap into delivering that straight away.

If we start fast, we will end fast, exhausted and numbed. The likelihood is we will have had very little awareness of others or ourselves during that day, because living frenetically means we lose connection with who we are and the world in which we live.

THE PLAN

To rebalance the speed, we are going to start slow.

SPEND THE FIRST TEN MINUTES OF THE DAY OUTSIDE WITHOUT DIGITAL DISTRACTIONS OF ANY KIND.

If it's impossible for you to get outside, stand by an open window, get some fresh air on your face and look out into the world.

The perfect place for these ten minutes would be sitting in a park or garden, but anywhere outside will give you the advantage we all need. Find a place that you are comfortable either sitting or standing and just be still for those ten minutes, breathing deeply with a smile on your face, observing and connecting with the world around you.

The peace and the space and the view of the skies help us plug in to the energy of the universe.

As you do so, you may notice certain thoughts come into your head. Just let them drift through without questioning them. What you will often find is that you will get a clearer perspective on who you are, and what is important to you right now.

THE PAYOFF

The moments when we first wake are precious. This is when we are most open to connecting to our essence, the planet and our core values.

If you make this a daily habit you will find that the connection you create in those first ten minutes of the day is much easier to sustain when things get busy. By making it a deliberate act you will find it easier to respond to the world and not just react. We will lose it for sure, but if we take a moment to breathe and smile and look to the skies, it will come back quicker and help us remember how fantastic this life really is.

SPREAD
THE LOVE

THE INSIGHT

Everybody on this planet is amazing. We all have things about us that make us unique and special, but often we lose touch with what they are and can therefore easily lose our shine.

Our brains are often more attuned to seeing the negative than seeing the positive, yet there are so many people around us who can be an inspiration to lift us up and help us make the best of every day. Meaningful human connection makes us not only happier but also healthier and helps us to live longer. A lack of it is more detrimental to our health than smoking and obesity. In short, we need it. Nobel Prize winner Daniel Kahneman found that our brains receive 20,000 individual inputs, or 'moments', every day. Most can be categorized as either negative or positive. The magic ratio for happiness is five positive moments for every negative one. In a *Today* interview, a successful, happy young man talked about his troubled background and difficulties in achieving at school. What changed his journey? When a grade-school teacher told him she cared and believed in him. This single encounter changed his life for ever.

PLUG IN

THE PLAN

TODAY, FIND ONE PERSON AND SHARE WITH THEM WHAT IT IS THAT YOU LOVE ABOUT THEM.

It can be anything at all. There are people in our lives who give us something special in often quite surprising ways. It may be the way that your partner leaves you notes around the house or in your bag when you leave for work. It may be the bus driver who always asks how you are doing with a big warm grin on his face. It could be your neighbour who put your bins out when you were on holiday. It could be a friend you haven't seen in over ten years, but has the uncanny knack of phoning you just when the time is right and listens to everything with such patience. It's the small details that count here, as it's the small details that add up.

THE PAYOFF

By doing this one simple thing, you will get a whole heap of benefits. First of all, you will program your selective attention to notice more wonderful things about everybody you come into contact with while living your life. If you perceive more positivity and brilliance, you will feel happier, connected and alive.

By sharing the love, you will also make deeper connections with those people that you have been appreciating, and deeper human connection has a direct benefit in helping us lead more fulfilled and happy lives.

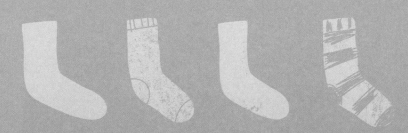

DRESS
THE SAME

THE INSIGHT

We can often obsess about how we look and the image that we portray, some of us spending as much as a year of our lives deciding on which clothes to wear. I have worked with people and indeed have friends who wear the same thing every day regardless of what they are doing, or how they feel. I used to think this was a strange bit of branding, but I have noticed more and more people extolling the virtues of this habit.

Steve Jobs was inspired by the workwear of Japan to simplify his wardrobe. Barack Obama told *Vanity Fair* that he adopted the 'only grey or blue suit' dress code because 'I'm trying to pare down decisions. I don't want to make decisions about what I'm eating or wearing. Because I have too many other decisions to make.' It is a modern phenomenon known as decision fatigue.

By eliminating a basic decision from their days, they are given more space to think about the big stuff.

THE PLAN

FOR THE NEXT FOUR DAYS YOU WILL WEAR THE SAME CLOTHES EVERY DAY.

It's worth spending some time thinking about what outfit is going to work best for you and which, indeed, you have enough items of to deliver four days of freshness. Then once you have decided, do not deviate from the path.

The time that you save in worrying about how you look can be used for purely pleasurable activities. Take longer over breakfast and consider your day. Have a proper conversation with loved ones before everyone scatters off to their business. Do some breathing and get yourself centred with a big smile on your face, knowing full well that today can only be great.

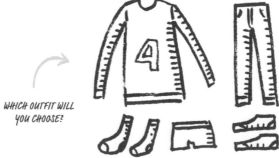

WHICH OUTFIT WILL
YOU CHOOSE?

THE PAYOFF

By taking that decision out of our lives we may just find that we are slightly more comfortable in our skins and have a little more time to think about what really counts.

Unless it's a very special occasion, I believe we should never dress for anyone but ourselves. If we feel good in who we are, that's all that counts. Mostly when we are dressing and taking too long deliberating, we are obsessing about how people will perceive us. How very tiring! Dress for you and enjoy it.

Of course after four days, if you have the desire to ramp up your look, then go nuts with it. If it's a part of who you are, there ain't no point holding back.

Slow
DOWN

THE INSIGHT

Life is getting faster. Our senses are overwhelmed by a constant bombardment of messages and the demand for decisions is escalating year in, year out.

With the increased connectivity we have through technology our inboxes are screaming for our attention while our friends are posting photos of their latest trip to the Gili Isles, which are too good to be missed. With so much going on, the conscious brain is prone to just shut down, so that our subconscious can filter out all the noise.

My good friend David Pearl and I set up Street Wisdom a few years ago. The principle behind it is that if you are in the right state, anywhere can be a source of inspiration. Therefore, we don't have to go to one of those bucket-list destinations like Machu Picchu to have a breakthrough. In short, any street can hold all the answers that you need, as long as you tune in. Thousands of people have experienced the benefits of Street Wisdom, now all around the world.

To help people tune in, one of our warm-up exercises is quite simply to get them to slow down. When people walk five times slower than their average speed, something amazing happens. They start to notice the world around them and indeed the world within them, because as we slow down we become more sensitized to everything.

THE PLAN

SPOT A TIME IN YOUR DIARY TODAY WHERE YOU NEED TO WALK SOMEWHERE AND PLAN IN SOME EXTRA TIME SO THAT YOU CAN TRULY SLOW DOWN AND ROLL AROUND IN THE EXPERIENCE.

Most of us are tempted to slow down a little, but this really needs you to slow down a lot. To push to the edge, see how slowly you can move and notice what happens when you do. Taking some deep breaths to slow the brain down will in turn help you slow the body.

If people look at you slightly strangely, just give them a little smile. Watch out for other people to whom you might ordinarily have been oblivious; when you slow down you often find that the most unusual of connections happen. In the words of superhero Bucky 'There is nothing in a caterpillar to suggest a butterfly,' until you slow down to find it. During Street Wisdom we have had the oddest of meetings when people almost pop out of the ether to tell us something we need to know. As we slow down, we connect more with ourselves and send out a more resonant and attractive energy. Sensitive folk are all around us and they will notice it and often come and play. Butterflies are all around us. Beautiful thought, huh?

THE PAYOFF

By quite simply slowing down you will notice so much more of the world and therefore become more awake. Many people who struggle with meditation due to the noise of their inner mind, find they can achieve peace incredibly quickly just by walking slowly, taking in big belly breaths, smiling and noticing what needs to be noticed.

Simply by taking a slow walk every day, you will find that you will become more conscious of who you are in a world that is moving fast. A clearer idea of how you interact with the world will make it so much easier to decide not to be carried away on an uncontrolled wave of busyness, but instead to plough your own furrow.

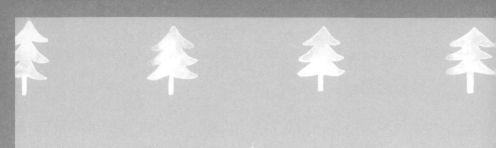

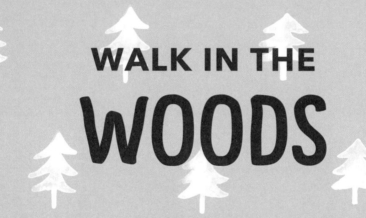

WALK IN THE
WOODS

THE INSIGHT

Japanese researchers have proven the medical benefits of shinrin-yoku, or forest bathing. One study shows that it reduces stress, anxiety and depression and therefore is helping reduce psychosocial, stress-related disease and also reduces blood pressure and boosts immunity.

Another study shows that it increases the body's NK cells, a component of the immune system that fights cancer. These levels remain increased for a week after a day-long dip in the forest bath, or for a month after a three-day soak. I love that.

We all know how good it feels to walk deep into a forest, breathe in the air that is thick with aromatic oils and soak up the energy. It's a place of magic, no doubt. We don't have to immerse ourselves for weeks into ancient woodland to feel the positive impacts of nature. All trees have the power to help us reconnect with ourselves and with the world around us.

THE PLAN

FIND SOME TREES AND WALK AMONG THEM.

The more trees the better, the older the better, the less polluted the better, but any trees will help. There are forty-four accredited shinrin-yoku forests in Japan, but I am sure you have one near you that may not have the stamp, but still has all the good stuff going on. Even in the most populated places there are trees nearby; find them and hang out.

When you're among them fill your lungs by breathing really deeply and notice how calming they can be. If you're a proper tree hugger now's the time to get down and dirty and wrap your arms around the trunks while breathing in the scent from the bark and immersing yourself in their auras. If you're not that full on, just love them for what they are: incredible living ecosystems. Take a leisurely stroll around them; then, when you have found a sweet spot, sit with your back against a trunk and breathe it in.

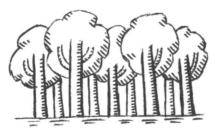

YOU DONT NEED TO BE IN THE COUNTRYSIDE TO FIND GREAT TREES; SOME OF THE BEST SPECIMENS ARE FOUND IN OUR CITIES

THE PAYOFF

If I have something that is troubling me or I notice that somehow I'm out of kilter, a walk in the woods will often put me right. It's hard to be obsessed by the modern world when we are surrounded by the ancient one. There is something truly primal about woodland as so much of this planet used to be filled with it. When trees surround us we ground our energy while also feeling connected to something so much bigger than ourselves. They act a little like a lightning rod for connectedness with the world.

Make trees your friends and you will find yourself waking up far more often. And remember some of the most amazing specimens are hidden within our cities. Go give them some love too.

LISTEN TO YOUR BODY

Centuries ago, people were more tuned in to their bodies. They listened more to how their bodies talked to them, letting them know about how the weather was changing, that they were missing something in their diet or, indeed, that it was time to stop working.

Few of us now make a living through our physicality, and even fewer need it to be a key tool of survival since we have warm houses with hot and cold running water. We have as a result become dominated by our mental energy rather than the physical, and yet we could learn so much if we listened more closely to our bodies.

When we are tuned in to our bodies and we have balance between our conscious and subconscious, listening to our bodies will help us understand some of our deeper processing and connectivity to the wider universe. Our intuition is precisely that. It is something that we feel in our bodies energetically that we then convert into knowing or understanding. If you listen more carefully to your inbuilt intuition, you will find it easier to wake up.

When there is something wrong with you and you are sick, the physical ailment is never without a connection to something else within your energy system that is also out of balance. If you tune in and ask your body what it is telling you, you may learn that there is something that needs to be addressed in your life that is creating this physical condition. For example, when we are stressed at work we are more susceptible to catching a cold. Other manifestations can be more serious.

I once worked with someone who had a persistent and distressing neck pain that no amount of physio, massage or osteopathy would shift. We spent some time on what was bothering her and found that she was angry that her clients weren't giving her more work, to the extent that she felt real resentment towards them.

When we dealt with that resentment by helping her turn around her beliefs and get more love in her, the neck pain disappeared for ever. There was nothing physically wrong with her neck; her beliefs were causing the problem.

When you tackle the area of your life that is out of sorts, so the ailment will often disappear.

Listen to your body and see what you can learn; in doing so you will wake up to a different consciousness.

FOLLOW YOUR
BODY CLOCK

THE INSIGHT

Our days are ruled by time. We awaken at a particular hour so that we can bathe, dress, eat breakfast and get to where we need to be when we need to be there.

As our time is dictated for us, we can often lose touch with choosing how we use our days.

When I write my books, I make sure there is nothing that I need to do but write. I make sure I am on my own and have no responsibilities for others. I disconnect from the outside world. I then follow the rhythm that feels right for me. Invariably my pattern becomes very different from my usual working routine. I get up very early and immediately start writing. By lunchtime I find I have done all I can do and spend the afternoons doing something physical to balance up all the creativity of the morning. I then go to bed ridiculously early, exhausted but happy, and let my mind make sense of the day. It's a natural rhythm for me and one by which I do my best work.

THE PLAN

THIS WEEK, TAKE THE OPPORTUNITY TO TUNE IN TO YOUR BODY CLOCK AND ASK HOW YOU MIGHT LIVE TO MAKE TIME WORK BEST FOR YOU.

I appreciate that some of the demands on our lives are less flexible than others and therefore we need to take into account jobs and schools and families etc., so you may need to do this at a time that you can manage more flexibility, for example in school holidays or at weekends.

When you've created the space just notice how you function at different times of day and for different activities. Eat when it feels right to eat and only eat the things that provide the necessary energy for that moment. Sleep when it feels right. Exercise when you need it. You may notice that it's different through the seasons, as well as for the varying activities in your life. It takes a few days to get into the rhythm, so just go with the flow until it clicks into place.

THE PAYOFF

Our modern way of living is not necessarily the most natural to us. The five-day working week is a recent construct. Sleeping once a day is also a relatively new habit when you look through history. By challenging some of these established structures, we may find a rhythm that suits us better.

Often autopilot kicks in because we are out of state. That is usually because we are fighting our energetic systems. When we work more sympathetically with our body clocks, we will find it so much easier to be in state and therefore to wake up.

Although we can't always dictate the times of our living, by tuning ourselves to work better, we can plan with more awareness and therefore give ourselves the best chance to be conscious more often.

POWER UP

CONSIDER TRYING THIS AT WEEKENDS OR DURING A HOLIDAY IF YOUR TIME DEMANDS AREN'T VERY FLEXIBLE

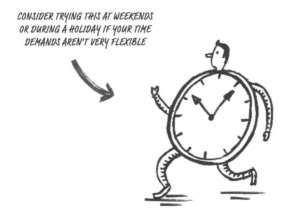

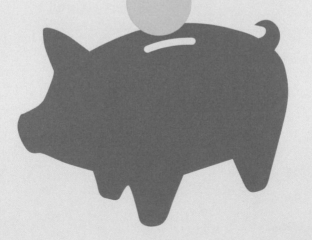

LIVE ON JUST

£5 a day

THE INSIGHT

If you are reading this book the chances are that you are amazingly affluent compared to much of this world. If you are concerned about raising your consciousness to lead a better life, it is unlikely that finding sufficient food and water and shelter are pressing issues for you.

It's sometimes easy for us to disconnect from some of the bigger and harder choices that others experience on a daily basis because we are lucky enough not to have to. We all know the statistics that are quoted ad nauseam: 1 per cent of the world's population owns 50 per cent of the wealth; 95 per cent of people earn less than £18,000 a year. Up to half of the food we produce globally is lost or wasted. Even if we saved one quarter of this it would be enough to feed 870 million hungry people in the world. We know things have gotten pretty badly skewed out there, but can we really appreciate just how well off we are?

When £5 (or $7.50 or €6.50) is your budget for the day, you have to consider carefully what you eat and drink, which purchases are absolutely necessary and which are not, and what is considered a real treat as opposed to something that just feeds a craving.

THE PLAN

TODAY WE ARE GOING TO LIVE ON £5.

Clearly, it would be impossible to include your mortgage, electricity, commuting costs etc. in this figure, but this is what you are going to spend to keep yourself alive.

It includes all sustenance, entertainment, hygiene, the lot. This will require some planning but will really help you tune in to what matters. You may consider walking to a meeting instead of taking the car or paying a bus fare; preparing meals in larger batches for freezing will save you chunks of change; entertaining yourself and friends at home is certainly going to be more cost-effective than lavish meals on the town. How can you make that money stretch?

Some find they can manage this quite easily for a day just by doing less. If that's the case for you, stretch it to a week . . .

THE PAYOFF

Although £5 a day may not seem like a lot, to others it's a fortune. Restricting our opportunities to spend by having such a fixed budget means that we have to really understand what counts and what doesn't. We will see the value in what we have already.

Most of the time we are cushioned from tricky decisions because we know they're not that important to us when we have abundant choice. When that choice is limited, and it becomes a little more painful, we have no option but to be more conscious of who we are and how we are living. Although this may be an uncomfortable wake up for some, it can also be an amazingly liberating experience.

TUNE IN

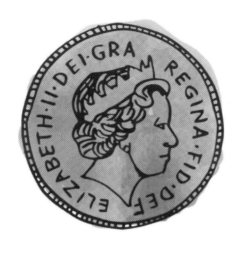

THERE ARE
PEOPLE WHO
HAVE MONEY . . .

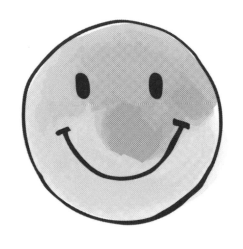

. . . AND THERE
ARE PEOPLE
WHO ARE RICH.

Coco Chanel

WRITE A
SONG

THE INSIGHT

Unfamiliar creative challenges will naturally engage us in a unique way. If we keep doing what we've always done, autopilot will stay firmly in control. If, however, we shake things up and push ourselves to self-express, we can't help but wake up.

Writing something that has no restrictions or rules and is innately personal helps us click into a different level of focus and presence. The best artists, musicians, dancers have an ability to drop into a space that gives them real depth of attention and a highly sensitized state, compared to the numbness of autopilot.

THE PLAN

YOUR CHALLENGE THIS WEEK IS TO WRITE A SONG.

We are all innately creative and I believe we all have amazing songs within us. My son, Harvey, writes songs constantly. He is ten and has yet to learn that we should find it difficult or leave it just to the talented. You don't have to be musical to write a song, you simply need to be able to hum a tune and put a few words to it. You can start with a rhythm, a lyric, or a riff, whatever. It's a game to play, not a tax return.

One of my friends is a songwriter and he always starts with a simple idea and builds around it. By the end, that starting point may be discarded, but no matter; it got him going. Some of these songs will not work and they will sound comical, but some of them will have genius within them and will fill your soul when you sing them. If you feel compelled, record it into your phone or, even better, sing it to someone you love.

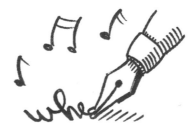

THE PAYOFF

Creative acts are as necessary for humankind as food and water. Often our creativity is stifled but it can never disappear. By having some fun with it on a project that has no pressure, we can see how brilliant that genius can be and realize it can also get it wrong.

Experimentation is the fuel of life. Trying things out and seeing how they work is what we should be doing every day, rather than doing the things we know are safe. Little experiments with our creative side keep us awake and make life spectacular.

YOU CAN START
BY SCRIBBLING DOWN
SOME LYRICS HERE
IF YOU LIKE

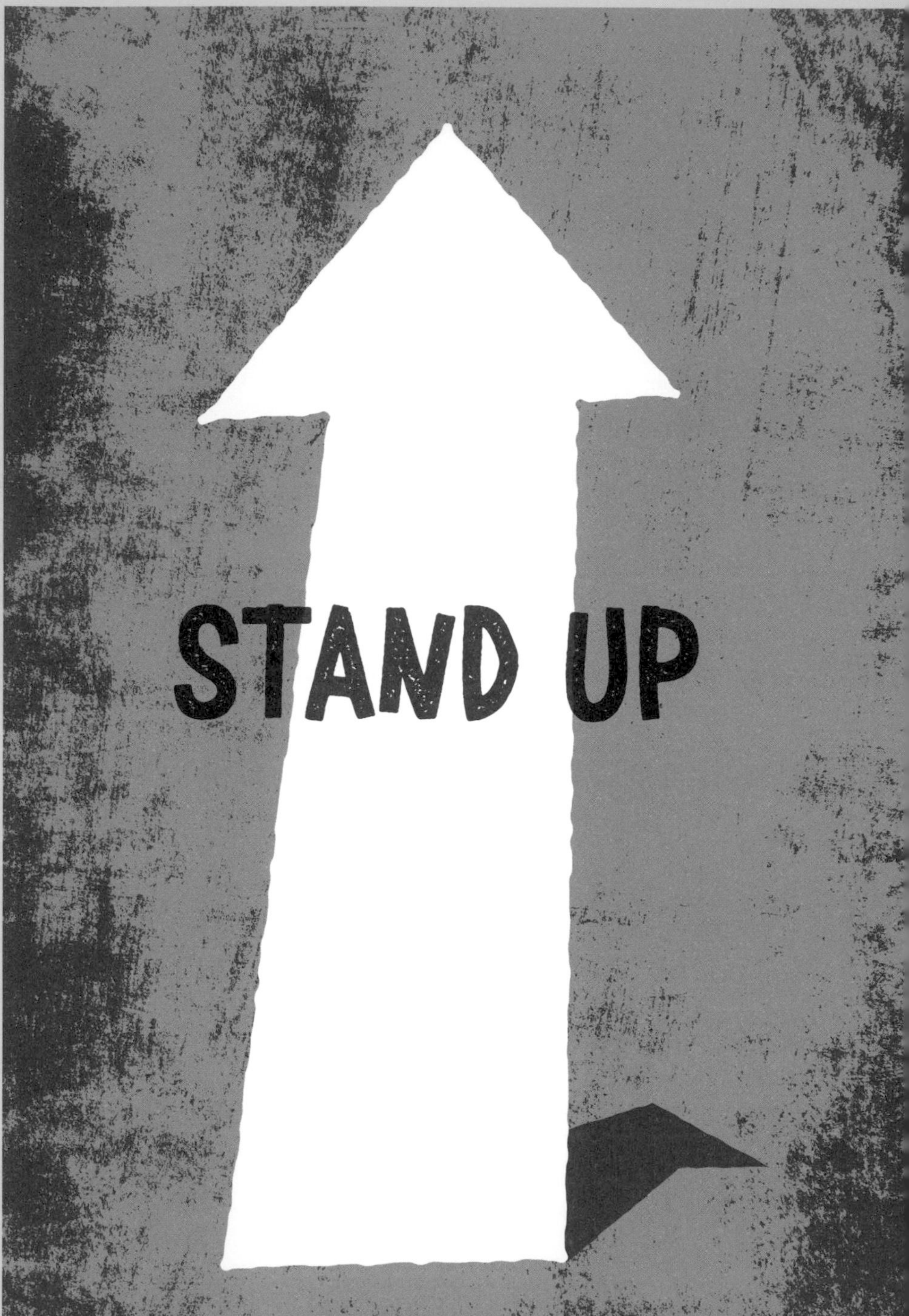
STAND UP

THE INSIGHT

One hundred years ago, only 10 per cent of us had sedentary jobs.

Today it's 90 per cent and it's becoming a big issue for our health and our energy. More people will die from diseases caused by lack of movement than from smoking this year.

When we don't move much, autopilot takes over, as being sedentary is where our subconscious brains feel most comfortable. If you want to wake up, move!

THE PLAN

THIS WEEK WHEN YOU ARE WORKING, BE THAT IN AN OFFICE OR IN YOUR HOME, SPEND AS MUCH OF YOUR TIME AS YOU CAN STANDING UP.

I am standing as I write this and I find it really helps my energy and focus. At my company, Upping Your Elvis, we often hold meetings while out walking; they are far more productive and much more fun, plus we get to see squirrels.

Some folk find that smart watches that monitor your movement are great ways to make sure you're not static for too long. If that works for you, then great. Do what you must to to get a wriggle on and not slump at a desk.

THE PAYOFF

Small amounts of regular movement help us keep the conscious brain firing. We all process kinaesthetically and therefore find it much easier to think when our bodies are fluid. I have a stand-up desk in my office and it has made an enormous impact on my work. I will never sit down to think again. The benefits of standing include reduced levels of fatigue, tension, confusion and depression, and more vigour, energy, focus and happiness, all of which will make it much easier for you to be awake for much more of the day.

_____

_____

_____

_____

_____

_____

_____

_____

_____

_____

_____

_____

SAY
YES

THE INSIGHT

As time goes on we start to make an internal map of what is wrong and what is right, and what is in and what is out. This map resides in the subconscious and helps autopilot steer us through the thousands of daily decisions that we have to make. This is an efficient part of our design because it means that we don't have to decide on every little thing we do each day, but instead we repeat what we have done before.

The danger with this process is that we become so deeply habituated that we don't even notice the wonderful opportunities of today as we are blinkered by the map of yesterday. I was inspired as a teenager by the book *The Dice Man* by George Cockcroft (under the pen name Luke Rhinehart). The book follows a character who makes all his decisions by rolling dice and then is committed to following them. By removing his need to make choices he undergoes an extreme transformation and certainly feels more alive as a result. It may be an extreme solution, and impractical outside fiction, but the insight is a good one.

THE PLAN

EACH DAY THIS WEEK SAY 'YES' TO SOMETHING THAT YOU WOULD NORMALLY SAY 'NO' TO.

It may be something as simple as going to lunch with folk at work that you wouldn't usually socialize with. It may be that instead of walking past the cinema as you do most days, you pop in, grab a little popcorn and enjoy the matinee. Sometimes the doleful eyes of the child struggling with their maths homework at 7 p.m. after a long hard day is just the invitation for help that we should take.

I tend to find that the best things to say yes to are the ones that create a strong reaction in me. That reaction could be excitement, surprise, nervousness or even rebellion. It doesn't matter as long as it wakes us up.

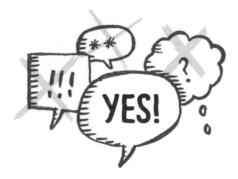

THE PAYOFF

There are opportunities around us every single day to which we are blind. By saying yes instead of no for a change, we open ourselves up to new avenues of life and therefore have to be more conscious, aware and awake as we engage in them.

It is always easier to say no than yes. Yes requires an openness and generosity and a no keeps things just as they are. Yes involves risk and no does not. Yes requires effort whereas no requires none. One little extra yes per day can be all we need to nudge ourselves to wake up and to reconnect with this world of possibility, and who knows who we may meet as a result?

See also Just Say No (page 216).

REALLY FEEL IT –
Emote
LIKE ELVIS

THE INSIGHT

Emotion in the workplace has been tainted by the 'let's be professional' posse. It would appear that they believe being emotional is a weakness and weak people do not win. That is bullshit.

Emotions are what make living an enriched experience. They help us understand what is going on in our world and how we interact with those around us. The twenty-first-century fad of bottling up emotions so that we can seem in control of them has taken its toll on many lives. Every time we bottle something up we are just creating a little minefield for the future, where at random they will explode, much to our surprise.

During a workshop in my home recently, a fire broke out in a downstairs room. By the time I got to it, it was absolutely raging. It was one of the scariest things I have ever seen. Fortunately, we had a large fire extinguisher in another room with which I was able to quell the flames. The fire fighters arrived to damp it down, I carried on with the workshop and all seemed fine. My wife was away that week and when she came home four days later, once I'd finished our programme, we sat and talked about the week. From nowhere I had this surge of emotion and was flooded with tears and shaking shoulders; the whole nine yards. The anguish and fear I had experienced in the fire had all been bottled up and it wasn't until my wife was home that I felt safe enough to let it go.

Emotions not dealt with will come back to haunt us physically, mentally, emotionally and spiritually. So we're going to get them out and love every second of it.

Do not apologize for crying. Without this emotion, we are only robots.

Elizabeth Gilbert, *Eat, Pray, Love*

THE PLAN

This week, when you notice that you are feeling an emotion of note (i.e. one that grabs your attention), instead of tucking it away and just powering through, truly engage with it.

Find space where you are comfortable, close your eyes and take a deep breath and properly feel that emotion. If it's a happy one you will notice that you quite naturally smile. Equally a sad emotion, when engaged with, most naturally will bring some tears. A proper blub is good for us and nothing to be ashamed of.

Do whatever you need to do to express emotion and notice how you feel as a result.

Huge caveat: there is a health warning with this. When other people are with you, remember that they might not be so cool with you expressing emotions, because largely they feel uncomfortable doing so themselves.

Laugh (or weep) alone until you feel that you have mastered the technique, and then you can start enjoying them with somebody else.

THE PAYOFF

By dealing with emotions in the moment, you will
find that you will be a lot more connected to yourself
and what is going on. A positive emotion fully
embraced just gets bigger. A negative emotion fully
experienced eventually dissipates and leaves you
free. By feeling them properly you will also notice
that your mind will quieten, which will help you be
in the moment and be more awake. Emote and
Wake Up!

A LITTLE
HOLIDAY
FROM BREAD
AND DAIRY

THE INSIGHT

There are certain staples in the Western diet that we would hardly ever question, bread and dairy being two of the most common. Ninety-nine per cent of American and European households buy them every week and consume them daily.

Cow's milk is meant for baby cows. Cows have a very different digestive system from us. Our bodies find dairy products pretty hard to digest. We buy them in part because mass marketing and commerce have led us to believe that they represent the easiest way for us to take in calcium, essential for the health of our bones and teeth. In fact, plant-based foods like broccoli, chard, kale, almonds and figs do a much better job. Bread has a similar story: the industry has moved a million miles from the simple origins of a handmade loaf of wholegrain flour, water and salt which would provide us with the sustenance and nutrition our bodies need. Now I am not suggesting that bread and dairy should never be eaten, but ingesting too much of them does have an adverse impact on our energetic state.

THE PLAN

CUT OUT DAIRY AND BREAD FROM YOUR DIET FOR FOUR DAYS. IT'S THAT SIMPLE.

No sarnies, no cappuccinos, no focaccia, no pizza, no yoghurt or toast. Hey, you know the list. For four days all of these are off the menu!

Now for some people this will seem like a terrible hardship, but I promise it isn't. It may take a little bit more work, but you can find amazing nutrition that doesn't involve either of these food groups. I eat a lot more fresh vegetables and fruit salads. Rice dishes and noodles are particularly good when hunger hits. Soups and stews can provide better comfort than any toasted sandwich. It is worth carrying some nuts and seeds with you, so that if you do get a little weak it will prevent fainting until you find a place that can serve you some proper food.

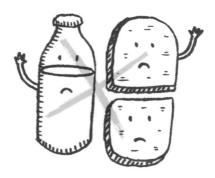

THE PAYOFF

When I first did this I was amazed how much bread and dairy I was eating and how unaware I was of it. I found it particularly hard to travel around Europe while not eating bread, especially in countries like Italy and France where meals on the hoof are traditionally white and floury.

What I also noticed was that I had more energy and I felt more connected to my body when I eliminated them. I have since added back a little bread, maybe once a week, but when I do eat it I choose locally made spelt sourdough over mass-produced fluff balls. With dairy, I find milk doesn't fit me at all, but of course a piece of stinky cheese on occasion lifts the soul so much the body doesn't care.

Give it a whirl and see what you learn about your body.

BE
SOMEONE
ELSE

THE INSIGHT

Who we think we are is who we become. All of life's rich experiences are little nuggets of insight that can potentially frame who we are.

The way we interpret those nuggets will shape both how we see ourselves and our identities. Unless you spend much of your life gleaning feedback from all those people around you, it's impossible to get a true perception of who you are and, even with the feedback, it's likely to be warped.

No one's identity is entirely fixed – human chameleons, we are all adept at modifying our behaviour according to the circumstances we find ourselves in – and when you couple that with the fact that we are constantly evolving as we live, grow and experiment with our personality, it's very easy for us to believe we are someone we are not. So, as we can flex like jelly on any given day, why don't we just push the boundaries of who we think we are?

THE PLAN

TODAY, BE SOMEONE ELSE.

Spend some time thinking about who it is you would like to be. The best characters are those that give us something back. Maybe you'd like to play with a little extra mischief, maybe a little extra drama, maybe some more flamboyance, or maybe just a little bit more 'I don't give a shit'; as long as it gives you a kick, it's worth a play.

It could be a made-up character, one from a film, or book, or someone from your past.

Imagine their lives and how they react to the world, while playing out some scenarios in your head. How do they carry themselves? What would they wear? What would they like to eat and drink? What are their favourite expressions? Get inside their skin a little in preparation for stepping onto the stage.

It may well be that this act is hard for you to keep up for long, in which case you should identify a moment in your day for you to become that person – maybe on the way to work would be a good time to experiment, or when you go shopping or for lunch. If their character fits well, wear it for longer and see what happens as a result.

THE PAYOFF

Our personalities are not fixed. We are flexible in who we are and how we present ourselves, and yet often we feel quite trapped in our own skins.

By playing with different personalities we might find there are aspects of ourselves that have been underplayed, which has resulted in us losing some of our shine. By bringing these to the fore and celebrating them, we can feel more alive and wake up to who we truly are.

It's hard to take ourselves too seriously when we're putting on a show. Let's enjoy the fact that we can stretch ourselves and bring a little more personality to all that we do.

PLUG IN

Journal

THE INSIGHT

When the pace of life is too fast we often don't get enough time to ourselves for reflection. Reflection is how we make sense of our experiences. Without time and space to do that, perceptions get warped and the connection we feel with our lives can become blurry.

By writing things down we clear our minds of some of the noise, we slow our brains down and we change our relationship with the things about which we write. When things are written on a page it changes our perspective, compared to when they are in our heads, swimming around like goldfish. This disassociation can give us power over our thinking almost like no other.

THE PLAN

EACH MORNING THIS WEEK, FIND A SPACE TO WRITE YOUR JOURNAL.

As near to when you wake is best as our minds are clearer and hence more creative then. Begin writing and just freestyle; don't worry about grammar or syntax. All you need is some paper and a pen, a cosy spot that is quiet and good for a ponder. Bed is a good, comforting place, even better if you have prepped the night before with pen and paper to hand and start writing as soon as you wake. Close your eyes, take a deep breath so you feel truly present and then write down anything that comes into your head.

Don't edit yourself, just let it flow. Some of the things that you write may be absolute nonsense; some things might not be true and some things might sound pretty dumb. Don't worry; just keep on writing.

Once you have written for a good ten minutes, take a moment to pause. Read it through if you like but if you do, make no judgement on its quality; we are not expecting Proust here. Just mull over what you have created.

THE PAYOFF

By creating some time for yourself to connect with what's going on with you in this amazing world of ours, and by giving yourself the chance to self-express in a way that is not critiqued, you will find you are more clear, grounded and dangerous as a result. I say dangerous because most of the time we are a little like a beautifully built fire that has yet to be lit. It may look great and have wondrous potential, but it's pointless. Clarity gives edge, and edge helps us become way more shiny.

Checking in with yourself provides the kindling that helps you light the fire every day. It guarantees that you focus your time and attention on what matters and not just on what seems most pressing. You'll also find that, when you listen to your subconscious and its creative outpourings, you will find it easier to think in new and innovative ways to explore all aspects of your life.

STEAL BACK
TIME

THE INSIGHT

Far too many of my clients seem to have no control of their own time. Much of the blame lies with shared diaries, or at least the bad use of them.

If you're not in control of your time you are not in control of your life and it becomes super easy just to switch off and live on autopilot as you bounce from one meeting to the next, never really having to take responsibility for any of them. It is a comfortable way of letting the days drift by, but it's certainly not the ticket to an awakened state and a life more extraordinary.

THE PLAN

EACH DAY THIS WEEK I WANT YOU TO STEAL BACK SOME TIME FROM YOUR DIARY.

It might mean you cancelling meetings or fabricating new ones that aren't actually happening. You might seek favours of friends so they pick up the kids. You may decide that this week the house doesn't need to be spotless and that its Thursday clean can just slide a little. Perhaps just before that business dinner you'll feel a little bit fluey and decide it's better for all if you don't pass on any potential germs.

Use your creativity and find a few spaces that you can enjoy.

The key to making this work is to make sure that you do not fill the spaces with anything other than stuff for you. You can do anything with that time, as long as it fills your soul with joy, or helps you connect more to yourself and the world. There is no point in stealing time if you let it be repossessed. Keep it, make it yours and relish the freedom and space it offers you.

THE PAYOFF

When we act more consciously to decide how we spend our time we naturally create space to move from autopilot into a more awakened state. By doing so over one week you will realize how much of your time seems to fill automatically, and how much of it is wasted as a result.

Be ruthless with your commitments and then when you do give your time, give it generously with full attention and focus and you will find that you have started to wake up more and more every day.

LOST IN MUSIC

Throughout the 1990s a psychologist called Alf Gabrielsson collected accounts of 'strong experiences related to music'. Here is one:

I was filled by an enormous warmth and heat. I really swallowed all the notes that were streaming out in the air, not a single note, effect or sequence missed my hungry ears . . . I was captivated by each of the instruments and what they had to offer me. Nothing else existed! I was dancing, whirling and really gave myself up to the music and rhythms, overjoyed – laughing. Tears came into my eyes – however strange that may seem . . . Before[,] I was in a very bad state. Depressed. It was during the most critical time ever in my life. I found it hard to get on with people and had to really exert myself to be able to get to grips with things. Afterwards I was bouncy, giggling, lively and filled with deep joy . . . it was so bewildering that it almost felt as a salvation.

Powerful stuff.

BE LOST IN
MUSIC

THE INSIGHT

Listening to music has a huge impact on the way we feel. It can synchronize our brain rhythms and therefore directly influence our emotions. When we listen to music we know and we love, our brains release dopamine, as they would if we were to take opium. Trippy.

Bob Marley was one man who understood the power of music very well: 'One good thing about music, when it hits you, you feel no pain.' It is a great healer. Not only that: when we listen to music the soundwaves impact every cell in our bodies, giving us a whole body massage to the unique rhythm and pitch of that tune. Music takes you on a journey like no other, but too often we just let it wash over us without fully engaging. It's often a part of the background noise, as opposed to something that we get properly lost in.

THE PLAN

For the next four days choose one piece of music that means something to you and sit in a place where you can properly soak it up. Eliminate all distractions and listen to it in as high a quality as possible. Notice where it takes you physically, mentally, emotionally and spiritually. Feel those soundwaves surround you and just let go. My favourite pieces of music evoke deep, emotional reactions. Some take me back to a very particular time and place; a moment that is somehow amplified beyond my daily experience. More often, though, I love music for the journey that it takes me on. If it's a piece that I can best appreciate only on my own in a quiet room with my eyes closed and the volume jacked to just the right level, then I know it's something that somehow touches me in a magical way – those are the pieces that I want you to play with. For me right now, I can't get enough of Sufjan Stevens. I put on Carrie & Lowell and off I go . . .

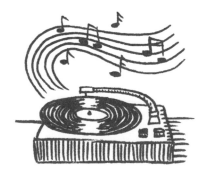

THE PAYOFF

Music is most often used to regulate our emotions. When we are in a bad mood it can get us out of it, or allow us to wallow in it. It can accentuate what we are feeling or help dissipate it. Regardless of where it takes us, it can help create dramatic swings in how we are feeling.

By immersing yourself fully in a musical experience you will notice that your emotions will be heightened and your imagination primed. This state can be a wonderful anchor to connect back to consciousness and to leave the world of busyness behind. In five minutes you can feel as if you've been to a spa for an hour and can come back rejuvenated, with a much clearer sense of how you want this day to be, ready to experience more shine.

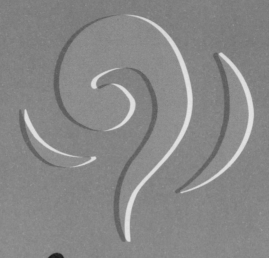

Make
A CUP OF TEA

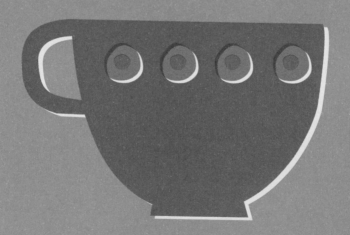

THE INSIGHT

When I asked a friend once about his top tips for properly being present in the moment he said: 'When you do the washing-up, do the washing-up.'

What he meant was that when we are doing menial tasks we often become lost in a world of imagination and conjecture. We aren't living in the now but imagining the future and indulging in the past. Our minds love to fantasize about what we're going to do next weekend, or how we should have told the boss exactly what to do with this week's report. Autopilot is in full control at that moment and therefore we are neither awake nor aware.

TUNE IN

THE PLAN

We are going to do one of the simplest tasks with absolute focus and awareness. We are going to make a cup of tea: Ceylon, Earl Grey, builders', green, dandelion or whatever tickles your taste buds.

Simply tune in to the moments that help make it.

Notice how your arm moves towards the tap.

You turn on the tap.

The water flows.

You move the kettle to fill it.

You turn off the tap.

You flick the switch (or light the gas).

You cross to a cupboard and open the cupboard door.

You select a cup and carry it to the kettle.

The kettle comes to the boil.

Your fingers lift the tea bag and drop it into the cup.

You pour the water and watch as the tea infuses, leaving it for as long as is necessary.

You carefully lift out the tea bag and add milk or lemon, if required (hopefully, no sugar).

The tea is made.

Before you lift the cup, take a moment to notice what you have just done.

Remain in the present. Notice how you lift the cup – lift it with as little effort as possible – notice your feet on the floor, drop your shoulders, smile.

Savour your tea.

Drink as if this is your first and your last cup of tea.

Repeat during the day and at any time in your life.

THE PAYOFF

If we can be fully conscious and awake when we are performing habitual actions, then we are retraining our brains to be present more often during our day.

Anything we do with full focus can be an enriching experience, so experiment with other activities that may feel like chores and see if you can use them to remember who you are. When we spend our lives imagining our futures and reliving our pasts, we cannot be connected with the now and so are running on autopilot. We must learn to wake up when doing things that would ordinarily be mundane, so that when we are doing things of real importance we can flick the switch on so much more easily.

WHAT TYPE OF TEA WILL TICKLE YOUR TASTE BUDS?

WHAT I
LOVE/HATE
ABOUT ME

THE INSIGHT

Most of us are far too self-critical and we listen far too much to the little voice in our heads. There is always a reason why we are not perfect, good-looking enough, smart, good, fit, funny etc., etc., and we can spend our whole lives looking for evidence to support it. If you look hard enough, of course, it will be there.

That life sucks. It is driven by the subconscious, which has an inbuilt negativity bias and therefore can only see the bad. It has been developed as a survival technique, but, as we know, in modern society spotting the danger in everything is no longer helpful.

Many years ago I went on holiday alone to Mexico. It was a pivotal moment of my life when I decided to find some space to think about who I was and who I wanted to be. As part of my exploration I learned that, in order to be fully present and connected, I needed to embrace my shadows as well as my light.

THE PLAN

On the space overleaf write all the things you love about yourself. Really relish this experience. Luxuriate in it. So many things about you are unique and special and make you who you are.

And then on the right, write down all the things that you hate about yourself. This is where you can twist the knife and spew out the vitriol. We all have it in us, so let's be truthful.

Once you have completed these two lists, spend a while looking at them and really soak them up. This may take some time but your challenge is to learn to love all aspects of both lists and to appreciate that, good or bad, they are what makes you who you are. Over time, in my workshops this process adopted the title 'Embracing My Arse'. This quite simply happened because of my inherent childish humour (also incongruously part of my 'arse'). The title makes me smile every time and hence speeds the acceptance process along the way. Call it what you like, but let's veer towards keeping this exercise a gigglesome one.

THE PAYOFF

When we embrace our shadows and realize that our foibles and imperfections are what actually make us who we are, then those voices go quieter and we have a chance to shine more brightly. When we love who we are, our connection to this life becomes such that we cannot help but be more conscious and awake. For most of us this is something we need to revisit constantly, but it is well worth the effort as it holds real liberation.

Happiness can only exist in acceptance.

George Orwell

THE THINGS I *LOVE* ABOUT MYSELF

THE THINGS I *HATE* ABOUT MYSELF

SUNRISE
OR
SUNSET

THE INSIGHT

When we all lived off the land and our families depended upon the weather for a good harvest, we were deeply connected to the planet as our fortunes directly correlated to it. We would rise with the sun and retire at dusk, adjusting the timing of our lives as the seasons unfolded.

Surprisingly, there were areas in France where, less than 200 years ago, people would still hibernate in the winter. They would literally change their living patterns as earth orbited the sun.

Nowadays, for many of us it's very easy to become disconnected from the world. We can cosset ourselves from the weather, have artificial light in the darkness and pretty much exist regardless of what is going on outside. This disconnection from nature robs us of the awe and wonder we can discover outside our windows every day. By rediscovering it, we have a chance to wake up.

PLUG IN

THE PLAN

This challenge is to be outside once a day, sitting quietly, at either sunrise or sunset (or, if you want the double whammy, both). When you do so, notice how it feels for the world around you to go from light to dark or dark to light.

Take your time and enjoy an event that happens every day, day in and day out. Sunrise and sunset are a constant in our lives and are not affected by events. Like time and tide, it is something that, for now at least, we can rely on. It's rare that we get to stop and fully appreciate the changing of night to day or day to night, and yet it is fundamental to the very pulse of the earth.

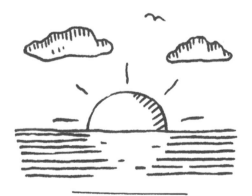

CONSIDER THE BIGGER PICTURE WHEN
WATCHING THE SUNRISE/SUNSET. ARE YOU
MAKING THE MOST OF WHAT YOU HAVE?

THE PAYOFF

When we consider that sunrise and sunset are governed by how the earth orbits the sun and spins on its axis, it helps us also to consider where we sit in this universe.

We are like specks of dust on the wind and yet get to hang out in the most beautiful and wondrous places where everything works in exquisite harmony. The chances of the atmosphere here being able to support life, and that it has flourished as it has, are so small that I can't help but wonder as to how we are doing. Are we really making the most of the gifts we have received?

Such a perspective helps us resist the constant attraction of autopilot and reminds us that to make the most out of this extraordinary life, we need to wake up.

There's a sunrise and a sunset every single day, and they're absolutely free. Don't miss so many of them.

Jo Walton

FIGHT THE
Amnesia

THE INSIGHT

The reason we spend so much of our time on autopilot is that the subconscious is very good at taking over our brains unnoticed. In those moments, we have amnesia. When I spend chunks of time gazing out of the windows of planes and trains and taxis, I often have no memory at all of time passing. I am so lost in my thoughts that I have no awareness that autopilot is on and I am in a state of dreaming.

We may experience peak states of connected consciousness while swimming with dolphins, dancing up the Himalayas or sitting quietly with a friend. However, we forget that this state is also available to us every moment of every day. When we return to our busy, hectic, everyday lives, the amnesia takes over and once again autopilot kicks in.

Louis Oosthuizen, the South African golfer, used a simple little trick to get his focus back and stop his distracted brain undermining his performance. He placed a simple red dot on his glove and would focus his attention on it when he was about to swing. This helped him create the right state to perform well. It was so successful that it helped him win the British Open in 2010.

THE PLAN

TO REMIND OURSELVES OF WHAT IS POSSIBLE AND TO REMIND OURSELVES TO BE AWAKE, WE NEED A HELPING HAND; IN FACT, IN THIS CASE OUR OWN HELPING HANDS.

Today, either put your watch on the other wrist or draw a flower on your dominant hand (it will be wobbly, but don't worry!). Every time you notice the watch or the flower, take a moment to sit straight, breathe deeply and put a big smile on your face so that you connect with who you are in that moment and in that place.

It takes about a week for most of us to make this a habit. So if you enjoyed it for a day, keep going and soon it will be part of who you are.

THE PAYOFF

Every time the watch or the flower spikes your attention and sparks a moment of self-reflection, deep breathing and awareness, you will find that this will kick you into waking up.

The more you do this, the easier it is to go back to that awake feeling and the less time you spend away on autopilot. Simple structural reminders like this make a huge difference to fighting the amnesia and we really need them, as there are so many other influences such as television and social media that are designed to induce autopilot.

_____

_____

_____

_____

_____

_____

_____

_____

_____

_____

_____

DIGITAL

DETOX

THE INSIGHT

Nowadays, you can't read a newspaper without seeing another piece of research about how our lives are being impacted by technology and that we need to learn how to manage it better.

We know technology is essential to human advancement, and is vital to us being better custodians of this planet. However, humanity is easily distracted; therefore, our relationship with technology needs to be relearned. Every time we hear a ping or feel vibration we get a little release of dopamine in our brains, making resistance to looking at our devices futile, hence we end up with the current situation that we are checking our smartphones on average 221 times a day. Recent research found that 80 per cent of millennials look at their phones on waking; this addiction is a strong one.

As a result, our cognitive processing has become shallower and we have become so distracted that we play directly into the hands of the autopilot. Digital devices are the modern-day equivalent of tranquillizers. They instil a trance-like state almost immediately as they are anchors for our subconscious to take over. We must learn how to manage the machines, rather than let the machines manage us.

THE PLAN

You have a choice of two, depending on how far you want to take this. One is easy, the other slightly more demanding. The easy way to manage a digital detox is to turn off all notifications on all of your devices, which includes email, calendar, apps, everything. Your challenge then is to look at your devices only when the time is right and you decide consciously to do so.

Bob Geldof recently put a ban on morning emails at his super successful TV company, Ten Alps. Every email received gets a message saying that their query will be dealt with after 2 p.m. 'I employ these people to have ideas,' he says. 'What's the point in having a company of secretaries?'

Work out which part of your day is most useful for you to connect to the digital world and limit yourself to just those moments.

For those wanting to go deeper into the detox, I would challenge you not to use anything digital at all for four days and see how you feel as a result. That will be a proper de-digification.

THE PAYOFF

By managing the way you interact with the digital world you will take control of your attention and focus and therefore find it much easier to stay conscious and awake. Remember that those devices put you on autopilot, and therefore that you should use them only when necessary.

When I did the full disconnect I found the first couple of days felt quite taxing, but soon it became extremely liberating. My phone once broke on a business trip and I had no way of getting reconnected for over a week. It turned out to be rather fabulous and taught me that technology is our friend when we consciously use it, and not when it uses us.

WILL YOU GO FOR THE EASY CHOICE OR THE FULL DISCONNECT?

GIVE IT SOME

CHANT

THE INSIGHT

Sometimes the things that feel the weirdest are indeed the best. Chanting is a much underrated beastie in the West and yet has been the foundation of thousands of people's spiritual grounding.

Sound has been used since the start of time, both literally and metaphorically, to generate different moods in people. Whether you talk about the formation of the universe as the Big Bang or God's creation, both must have involved sound and vibration. Every cell in our body is vibrating constantly, and when we get them to work in harmony, it is a beautiful thing. (Sounds super hippie, but it is actually anchored in science.)

Chanting is practised all over the globe, including in Japan, much of Africa, Hawaii, Tibet, North America and Europe, and in various guises remains one of the more colourful aspects of most major religions. If it's that widespread, there must be something in it. It's been proved to help with anxiety and depression but, for me, it's a form of creative self-expression that's helped get me into the here and now and has put a massive grin on my face. It's not that I chant every day, but it's one thing that I always have in my pocket for when the time is right.

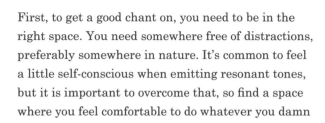

THE PLAN

First, to get a good chant on, you need to be in the right space. You need somewhere free of distractions, preferably somewhere in nature. It's common to feel a little self-conscious when emitting resonant tones, but it is important to overcome that, so find a space where you feel comfortable to do whatever you damn well want.

I am not a believer in a prescribed chant (although certain sounds have certain benefits, for sure). I personally like to see what noises come out, what sounds good to my ear and is feeling great to my heart. This isn't about nailing a perfect Gregorian chant, or even a tuneful 'Om mani padme hum', but getting your own sound into the world. Don't be afraid to experiment, throw out some sounds and see which ones capture your attention and are fun enough to keep repeating. Lose yourself in it until you feel it has taken you far enough.

If you're stuck, try some whaa whaa whaa whaa's, or some shucky shucky shucky shucks. I sometimes begin with some fucky fucky fucks until my head clears and more positivity is emitted.

No rules, just find what feels good and repeat.

THE PAYOFF

Once you make chanting your friend, you will find that it can take you to a different space very quickly. The resonance in your chest and head has a very particular effect, depending on which notes and sounds you throw out. When you hit the one that is right for you now, you can become extremely well connected with yourself and all around you, and profoundly awake in a very short time.

If you don't quite get to spiritual nirvana, fear not. Chanting often has the wonderful side-effect of setting up a right good giggle.

CLIMB A
TREE

THE INSIGHT

The simplest of pleasures are often the richest, and yet the way that we lead our lives means that we commonly detach from them. As we age, our lives naturally become more complex.

We have ever more and varied responsibilities, so cannot help but fractionate our attention. We rush from one task to the next, juggling our work and home lives, being with our families, getting the shopping done, taxing the car, preparing meals and organizing the kids. Even fun stuff like planning next year's holiday can leave us feeling dissatisfied. The more functional each action becomes, the more time pressured it feels. We have lost the twinkle in our eye.

As children we could find joy in pretty much anything; cardboard boxes provided hours of entertainment. We loved to escape into our own little worlds created through fantasy and the purest joy. This challenge will help us reconnect with that and help us feel more alive and exhilarated.

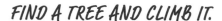

THE PLAN

FIND A TREE AND CLIMB IT.

Trees have been in existence for 370 million years, and with around 3 trillion mature trees growing in the world, each one certainly has a story to tell. Some scream out 'Climb me!' and some don't. Find an inviting and friendly tree that requires a little exhilaration to climb, but no extreme effort or life-endangering peril.

It's not about climbing the highest tree, just the one that appeals. And please climb within your limits or not at all. This exercise isn't for everyone.

If you do climb, don't rush it. Enjoy the smell of the leaves, the touch of the bark and the gradually changing view.

Most trees have a place to sit that feels just right. It's worth spending some time finding that place; you'll know it when you do. Now, take a deep breath and hang out there. Notice how connecting to nature it is and yet how disconnecting it is from the busy life we often lead. Notice also the difference in climbing up, to coming down; cats do.

If you feel drawn back to this tree, climb it again tomorrow. If not, find another one.

THE PAYOFF

By doing simple things that can fill our souls with childlike joy we reconnect both to who we are and to the planet on which we live. It's easy to believe that the only way to achieve a profound shift in consciousness is to do something big and bold like throwing in your job and walking the length of the Nile. I'm sure that such adventures are good for the soul, but they aren't everyday living. The simple stuff is what we can do, whenever it's needed, without the expense of plane tickets and malaria pills.

Tree climbing also lets us reconnect to who we once were. There is still a kid in each one of us and it's begging to play more and to not take life so seriously. By letting out the inner child we will find real joy in the simple act of living. We don't need more stuff; we often just need to lighten up and have a giggle.

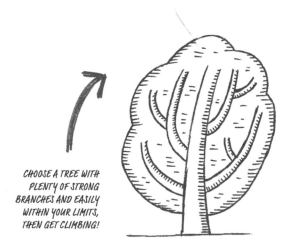

CHOOSE A TREE WITH
PLENTY OF STRONG
BRANCHES AND EASILY
WITHIN YOUR LIMITS,
THEN GET CLIMBING!

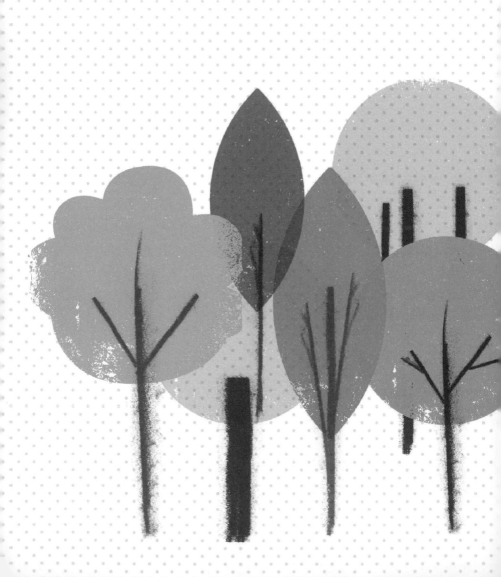

THE
SIMPLEST
PLEASURES
ARE OFTEN THE
RICHEST

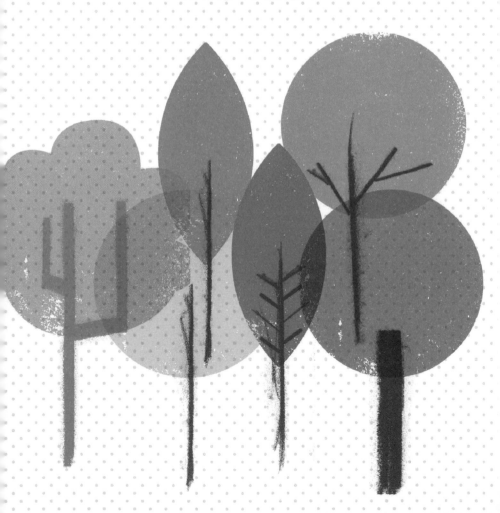

EAT WHEN
HUNGRY

THE INSIGHT

Some years ago I went to Thailand for a fasting retreat. I couldn't believe how good I felt as a result and have since been fascinated by our relationship with food and how it affects the way we feel.

There is plenty of research out there that suggests that fasting not only helps us stay in shape, but also aids brain function, increases energy, prevents type II diabetes, delays Alzheimer's and fights cancer. Powerful stuff. Hara hachi bun me (packs quite a pun in its translation) is the ancient Japanese Confucian teaching that instructs people to eat until they are 80 per cent full. More prosaically, it has been proven to help extend life expectancy in laboratory animals. Either way, it helps us be more aware of how much we are eating.

When we de-tune ourselves from what we put into our bodies and ignore what we need in favour of what we want, we eat too much and the wrong stuff. This induces a sort of dietary coma, which invites autopilot to the party.

THE PLAN

THIS WEEK I WANT YOU TO EAT ONLY WHEN YOU ARE TRULY HUNGRY, AND TO EAT ONLY SMALL AMOUNTS.

You may eat ten times a day if necessary, but by making the portion size smaller you start to realize what you absolutely need, rather than what you crave.

To begin with, it's common to crave junk food, but as you start to eliminate some of the toxins and your body becomes purer you will notice that the cravings start to shift. Depending on your physiology, the climate and even the time of year, your tastes will vary, but if you follow the regimen, you will be rewarded.

The fresher and the more raw you can safely make your food, the more enhanced your energy system will become. Often we confuse thirst with hunger, so drink plenty of water and obviously avoid refined sugar, caffeine and booze. Keep in mind food guru Michael Pollan's words, 'Don't eat anything your great-grandmother wouldn't recognize as food,' and all will be well. If you have or are susceptible to any eating disorder, you should not attempt this experiment.

THE PAYOFF

When we are more aware of what we need to fuel our system, we will make sure we put the right energy in to get the right energy out. Overeating and eating sugary foods will create a state in which it is very challenging to remain awake. Overeating numbs the mind and sugar overstimulates it; either way it kicks you out of balance.

By holding high standards for what you consume, you will naturally become more conscious and find it a key contributor to waking up.

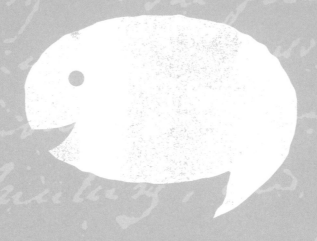

UNTOLD
Story

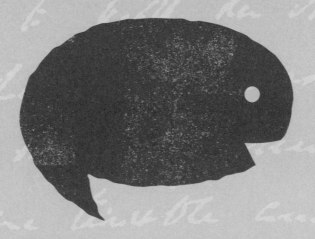

THE INSIGHT

I believe that we all have a story that needs to be shared. It's a narrative that explains both why and how we have become who we are.

Your personal story is one that you wouldn't ordinarily share, and yet we subconsciously return to our stories every day as a means to explain how we show up in the world. Much of our lives have passed without the chance of great reflection. It is difficult when you're busy to step back and appreciate experiences for what they are, and because of that these stories we tell about ourselves can grow into mythical beasts without us even realizing, yet they have a direct impact on how we live and how brightly we shine.

I know a girl who believed that being dumped by her boyfriend before her exams resulted in her not getting to the right university, not getting the best job, therefore not having the best life and therefore not trusting men for the rest of her days. Turns out the story isn't quite true as it got embellished by her in her head over time. It helped her make excuses, but not make an amazing life.

THE PLAN

This week think about a story you have never told. A story that somehow has a bearing on who you are today. Spend some time breathing deeply with your eyes closed just remembering the small detail of that story and reliving the energy of it. Once you have reconnected with that story, find somebody in your life that you trust and tell it to them. Just ask them to listen without passing judgement and explain that this is an experiment in connecting with your past, and as a result connecting more deeply with others.

Take your time. There is no rush. As you tell the story, notice any movement of energy in you and keep smiling, breathing and looking your friend in the eye. You may decide as a result of this experience to then tell the same story to other people in your life. As you tell more and more people you may find that the story changes. You might give certain aspects of the story greater emphasis than others. That's fine, it's your story.

You may decide that there are other stories that have more emotional resonance with you, and they are the ones that should be told. That's fine too. There is no right or wrong, but this sort of storytelling can help you find a deeper connection to what makes you tick.

THE PAYOFF

Our stories can act as liberators or incarcerators. The significance we place on them is often far greater than we are aware of, and by sharing them we can raise our consciousness and use them to help us pop out of our daily fogs. Some inhibiting stories when told become laughable and we realize they are just fabrications, thus setting ourselves free. Others help us understand more about who we are.

The space to reflect on important moments of our lives and to share them with somebody we care about can be deeply therapeutic, and if nothing else will help us all feel that little bit more alive. Too much of our time is spent focusing on things that are irrelevant. By telling your story you'll be focusing more on what counts. When we engage in what counts, we can't help but wake up.

DO SOMETHING NEW

THE INSIGHT

It is very easy to lead a life full of habit. We have our favourite sandwich shops, our favourite newspapers and our favourite seat on the bus. There is something warm and comforting about doing the same stuff day in, day out because we crave familiarity. We are led to believe that if we stick to the familiar routine in life the terrifying prospect of uncertainty will stay away.

The problem with living like this is that it triggers the autopilot. If we experience the familiar our subconscious brains automatically kick in so that our conscious brains can relax. In short, the more habituated our lives, the less awake we are.

The future will pretty much largely, for the important parts, look like it does today. So stop worrying about what might happen (because it most likely will never happen) and go find a lot of the brilliant stuff we are missing out on by doing the same old same old, every day.

Have some fun, experiment and try on a life of Technicolor. Who knows what shades will look the best on you?

THE PLAN

TODAY, DO SOMETHING NEW.

It can be anything at all as long as it seems a little more fun and exciting than the norm. It could be that you buy your lunch from somewhere new. It could be that you listen to some music you haven't heard before. It could be that you try that hobby that you've always been interested in. It could be simply striking up a conversation with a stranger. The important thing is that it's something new and different to you.

Often when facing a new challenge our caveman brains will kick in and see potential danger. Just breathe and smile and notice it for what it is: a normal fear reflex to uncertainty. When you are engaging in that new activity notice how your senses can be heightened, and that your awareness of where you are right now is slightly more resonant than usual. After engaging in new fun things it can be that we take a more liberating perspective into other aspects of our life that feel a little bit stuck. Use this perspective and shake things up; who knows what will happen as a result?

THE PAYOFF

A couple I know wanted to go away for the weekend but didn't have the budget. So, instead they stayed in their spare bedroom, where they'd never slept before, and just did touristy things in their home town. They felt like they'd had a complete break from the norm and woke up to more possibility.

Bringing new experiences into your life will make autopilot struggle to take control as anything new creates a more awakened state in us. By regularly breaking simple habits and trying something fresh, you will find it so much easier to be conscious and alive, and therefore be able to be more yourself and live a more extraordinary life. It's also addictive (in a good way).

What **NEW** things can you try today?

JUST
Say No

THE INSIGHT

To be in control of your life you must be up to saying no. There are constant demands on our time and our attention and unless we learn to manage them, we will drown. We love to help people and often feel that we gain a great deal of our purpose and meaning by doing so. But if we're not there for ourselves, how can we be there for anyone else?

Busyness feeds autopilot. To be conscious we need to find space, and therefore we need to learn to say no. Often, if we say yes to something we are not fully committed to doing, we subconsciously fuel inner resentment. We are not being authentic to ourselves. Shame and vulnerability researcher Brené Brown explains, 'Compassionate people ask for what they need. They say no when they need to, and when they say yes, they mean it. They're compassionate because their boundaries keep them out of resentment.' It seems like a paradox; agreeing to something feels like you are being compassionate to another person, but if it isn't authentic, it has quite the opposite effect.

THE PLAN

Each day this week, deliberately and consciously find something that you would usually say yes to, but in this case, say no. Don't do this out of spite or out of anger, but do it out of love for yourself. Choose something that you would ordinarily find it difficult to refuse, but feel deep down it is right to do so. Deliver your refusal with clarity and lightness. It doesn't need great explanation or justification. Keep it simple. Saying no to an ingrained habit that people assume you will do every day can be amazingly liberating. If you always put the kids to bed, maybe it's time you didn't. If you always make the office tea run, perhaps it's someone else's turn. If you always do the washing-up, maybe it's time to grab the tea towel.

When you have said no, notice how liberating it feels.

THE PAYOFF

When we say no to a responsibility that we would ordinarily accept, we have to be conscious. We are also building more time into our lives, so that we can be more awake. When we say no it gives us space to say yes to ourselves and to others with all our hearts, and not through duty.

See also Say Yes (page 134).

TUNE IN

DANCE

THE INSIGHT

I used to lead a team of the most extraordinary people. Most of us have had moments when we have found ourselves surrounded by folk who live life to a higher standard and therefore create magic beyond the norm, and this was one of mine.

When I tried to understand what it was that united the team, my analysis was found wanting. The only thing I could find that everyone loved to do (especially when together) was dance.

Many studies have shown how great dance is for us, not just physically but mentally, emotionally and spiritually, but frankly, you don't need to know the research as this is something nearly all of us have personal experience of. We know how good it feels when we put on just the right tune and lose ourselves in dance with complete abandon. Dancing is life and is a practice that unites all humanity.

THE PLAN

THIS WEEK FIND SOME TIME TO GET YOUR BOOGIE ON.

Sure, you can go clubbing or hit a party, but weirdly there is something also deeply satisfying about having a strut and a wiggle on your own.

Find ten minutes in your day, choose a tune that makes you tingle, crank it to ten and lay out some moves that bubble up from within, caring not one jot what anyone thinks. This ain't about looking good, or being cool, this is about shaking it out for the hell of it.

THE PAYOFF

To begin with it may feel a little strange to dance on your own, but once we overcome the internal judgements and the little nagging voices in our heads, it just feels good. When I am stuck and finding it hard to have fun because life feels just a little too serious, one of the best antidotes I know is to put on some Sly and the Family Stone to show me the way, and then my body has no choice but to join in.

Once you have mastered dancing on your own behind closed doors, feel free to break out some moves spontaneously as the mood takes you.

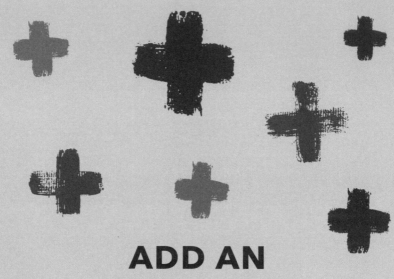

ADD AN
HOUR
TO YOUR DAY

THE INSIGHT

One of the most frequent comments I hear from people is that they are not living the lives they want because they don't have the time. It may be that they don't read enough, exercise in the way they'd like to or practise the piano as often as they should. Usually it is explained with doleful eyes that these things would absolutely change their lives but they are too busy to embrace them into their daily routines.

Time has many definitions, some controversial, others widely agreed upon. Relatively uncontroversial definitions are 'time is what clocks measure' and 'time is what keeps everything from happening at once'. Once we grasp the fact that time is a perception that we can control, we realize that when we don't have time to do something it's because it is not important enough to us. The ancient Chinese philosopher Lao Tzu explains: 'Time is a created thing. To say, "I don't have time," is to say "I don't want to."'

THE PLAN

THIS WEEK LET'S FIND OUT EXACTLY WHICH HOBBIES OR ACTIVITIES WOULD REALLY MAKE A DIFFERENCE TO YOU LIVING AN EXTRAORDINARY LIFE, AND THOSE WHICH ARE JUST MISSHAPEN DREAMS.

There is a little pain involved, but I think you'll find it will deliver multiples of pleasure.

For four days try waking up an hour earlier and do one of those things that you wish you had time for. Fully engage in that activity for sixty minutes, and enjoy the fact you're stealing some time to do something that could fill your very soul.

You could repeat the same activity for all four days or try a different one for each. The choice is yours. The key to this is to make sure it's something you feel you would love to do, not just something you feel you ought to do.

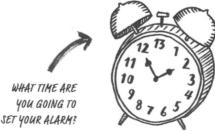

WHAT TIME ARE
YOU GOING TO
SET YOUR ALARM?

THE PAYBACK

At the end of the week you then will be able to deduce whether what you've been doing is something that you have to have in your life because you find it enjoyable and fulfilling, or whether it's not as important as an extra hour's sleep, in which case you can take it off your list.

Either way you will now be better informed about what you truly need in your life.

EXCITEMENT AND
Gratitude

THE INSIGHT

It is common for us to find life a blur and to disconnect from the highs and lows. The pace of life and our fractionated attention all contribute to the blending of our experiences.

To wake up we need to tune in to what is happening to us every day. Excitement is part of our fuel and makes us feel more alive. Gratitude has recently been researched extensively and has been shown to improve both sleep and positivity as well as physical and psychological health. It's a one-stop shop for getting us geared up to living a great life, for sure.

THE PLAN

EACH MORNING WHEN YOU WAKE UP WRITE DOWN THREE THINGS HAPPENING THAT DAY THAT YOU ARE EXCITED ABOUT.

Perhaps you are looking forward to catching up with a friend, anticipating the next chapter of a book you are enjoying, have made time to hit the gym or even finally have a chance to sit down with your boss and plan the next quarter.

Each evening, write down three things that happened that day for which you feel grateful. Take a moment to ponder the day and pull out the highlights. Did you have a proper chat with your daughter on the way to school, or land a new piece of business, or wake refreshed from a great night's sleep, or find that old mix tape (the very best mix tape ever made, ever), or finally finish *Infinite Jest*?

For some people, sharing these lists with their loved ones helps accentuate the emotions and makes the experience even more conscious. Try it and see for yourself.

THE PAYOFF

Every day is unique and special and every day can hold amazing experiences if we seek them out. When they all merge together it's hard for us to find those little nuggets of joy. By attuning ourselves to what we are excited by, we increase the chances that we will make them happen and will be energetically ready to actually be excited.

Gratitude is key to happiness and to breaking us out of autopilot. When we are grateful we naturally connect more to ourselves, to others and to the planet. When we take things for granted, we don't have the same moments that jolt us into consciousness as each moment can feel expected and too familiar. Gratitude, by definition, means appreciating the uniqueness of our experience more deeply and is therefore emotive; when it's felt, it creates a visceral reaction in us and helps us wake up with big smiles on our faces.

£50 MILLION

THE INSIGHT

People often hold themselves back from achieving their dreams by making up excuses. If only I were taller, prettier, better at maths; if I just could have gone to Harvard, sold my house at the top of the market, got that promotion, invested in snapchat, blah blah blah.

The truth is that we have everything we need now within our grasp to make our lives extraordinary. However, it is much easier to keep living the life that we lead now, and blame it on circumstances, than to step up and make the change, because with any change there is implicit risk and our caveman brains (see page 6) aren't too pleased with that. We therefore stay small and keep whining about our lives. Today will change that.

THE PLAN

I WOULD LIKE YOU TO IMAGINE THAT YOU HAVE JUST WON £50 MILLION.

You now have no limitations as to how you choose to spend your life. Close your eyes, take a deep breath and think about what it is that you will do with your life now. How will that money change you? Dream a little and get lost in the fantasy.

Our first impulses are often about where we live and our houses, our cars and our holidays, but I want you to explore a little beyond that as to how you would spend your days rather than your cash. When you have unlimited choice, how do you want to pass your time? What joys do you bring into your life when everything is possible?

Make a list of all the things you would do. Don't hold back; this is a time to dream.

THE PAYOFF

I often find when people carry out this exercise, when you dig deeper into how people want their quality of life to be, those things don't need £50 million; they can be achieved now. One of my clients explained that his dream would be to buy a farmhouse in Provence with an amazing view, to go there and write novels.

He then realized that his flat already had an amazing view and there was nothing to stop him from writing his first novel immediately.

Don't delay your dreams. Live them today and your autopilot will no longer fill your brain with fantasy, as your reality will be even better.

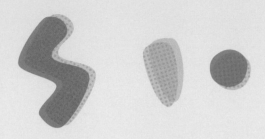

GROWN-UPS NEVER UNDERSTAND
ANYTHING FOR THEMSELVES,
AND IT IS TIRESOME FOR CHILDREN
TO BE ALWAYS AND FOREVER
EXPLAINING THINGS TO THEM.

ANTOINE DE SAINT-EXUPÉRY

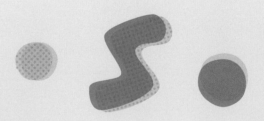

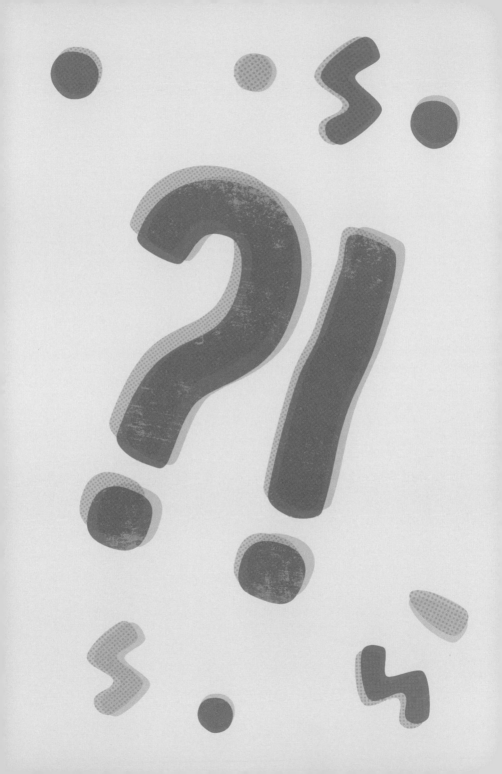

STARE AT
THE SKY

THE INSIGHT

The sky is constantly changing and is a marvel when we stop to notice it. Most of our lives are spent looking at our feet rather than the heavens.

Our vision tends to be locked on other people, where we are walking, the phones in our hands, so we miss what is above us most of the time. We cannot comprehend its vastness. Our universe is billions of years old and space is infinite. Just think how many people have gazed up at the same sky since the dawn of time, and lived such different lives from yours. An expansive view helps us recalibrate from the pace of life and reminds us who we are and where we are living.

PLUG IN

THE PLAN

FIND A NICE SPOT OUTSIDE WHERE IT'S COMFORTABLE TO LIE DOWN AND SPEND TEN MINUTES JUST WATCHING THE SKY.

There may be clouds that morph into shapes that capture your imagination; it may just be shades of blue that seem to stretch out beyond your grasp; it could be a night sky where all forms of twinkle are apparent.

Soak it up and notice where the experience takes you. If you do this regularly, you'll start to notice the beauty of the heavens more frequently.

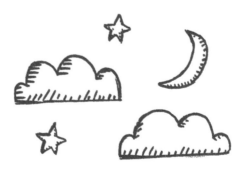

YOU COULD LIE IN A GARDEN OR A PARK,
OR MAYBE ON A ROOFTOP IF YOU'RE
FEELING ADVENTUROUS . . .

THE PAYOFF

We are so lucky to have such a humbling stimulus as
the sky above us every day. When we remember to
connect with it, it helps us overcome the amnesia so
that we can truly wake up to our place in the world.
It reminds us that we are part of something much,
much bigger, that the things that bother us are
largely irrelevant and that our time should be spent
on what counts and not what can be counted.

PLUG IN

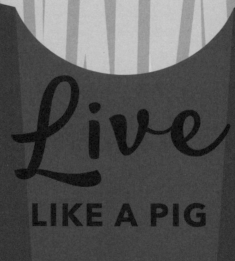

THE INSIGHT

I always encourage people to mess with these exercises to make them work even better for them.

In January 2016 thousands of people started cooking food from scratch for a week as part of The Great Wake-Up! project that inspired this book, with many having profound breakthroughs because of it. One person, however, said that because she always cooks food from scratch, for that week she would do the opposite. She ate fast food, stuff in tins, rubbish that was full of refined sugar and preservatives. Interestingly, she had one of the most profound breakthroughs of all those taking part in the exercise, as sometimes having a severely negative experience jolts us back to the positive. She felt lethargic, her skin became blotchy, she was bloated, she got headaches, and she got a really clear idea of why putting the right food into her body was worth all the effort.

THE PLAN

THIS WEEK, RATHER COUNTERINTUITIVELY, LIVE LIKE A PIG.

Eat ready-prepared meals, live like a slob, go on a bender (2 bottles of vimto and a packet of wotsits!), watch a whole box set, don't tidy the house . . . in fact, take the brakes off and live as if you just don't care about today or about tomorrow.

Do all those things that feel as if they are below your usual standards. For some, that might mean eating a doughnut; for others, it would be getting up late, dressing sloppily or having a beer at lunchtime (or all three). Relish dirty living and notice the difference that it makes to your level of consciousness.

Please do not attempt this exercise if you have issues with drugs, alcohol, eating disorders or other behavioural problems, as a trip back into the darkness is probably not what you need. For everyone else, live like a pig with full commitment until it repulses you.

THE PAYOFF

Sometimes, for us to be aware of how great every moment can be we have to make our situation just a little bit worse. When you talk to people who have made profound life shifts for the better, it is usually because life just got so bad that they had to make a change to pop back up.

For those of you who enjoy the pig living a little too much, imagine if this were how you lived your life every day for the next thirty years. How would you be then? What would you stand for? What would you have made of life's gift?

A little journey to pigdom ain't bad, but a life there has implications far beyond saving on vacuuming.

Pushing our standards below what we would usually consider acceptable can help us reconnect with what's important for us and make sure that in future we never ever, ever, ever let those standards slip again, because when we do we are automatically playing into the hands of autopilot.

OWN IT
- NO EXCUSES

THE INSIGHT

This life is yours and nobody else's. Although at times it can feel as if life is conspiring against us, the energy that we put out into the world is the energy that we get back, and therefore the life that you are leading right now is a result of how you show up in the world.

If everything seems hard and painful, maybe it's because you aren't living positively. If everyone around you seems flaky, often it's because we aren't clear enough about what we commit to in order to make our lives extraordinary. If we don't find enough love in our lives it's often because we don't love ourselves enough.

Regardless of the specifics of cause and effect, how we are dictates what we attract. Our world is our creation and not one that happens by accident.

Most events on this planet are far beyond our control, but the way we react to them is absolutely in our hands. We can all choose how we respond to the good, the bad and the ugly, and that choice will shape our quality of life.

We should never try to make the world work to our agenda but we should constantly strive to use its lessons in a fruitful way.

THE PLAN

THIS WEEK I WANT YOU TO OWN YOUR LIFE.

Notice when things happen that create a negative reaction in you. Notice when you make excuses to yourself, or blame circumstances for the fact that something is not quite perfect.

As you notice a negative emotion in your body, breathe into it so that it is fully experienced. Then ask yourself what it is that you are thinking that's making you react in a negative way. I recommend writing down in the space provided everything that is driving this reaction.

Ask yourself which of your statements are absolutely correct, and which are simply excuses to feel sorry for yourself. When you do this you'll find that a lot of your arguments are not justified at all, and therefore it's easy to overcome negativity. If there are some things that are irrefutable and still create a negative emotion, ask yourself how you might embrace this feeling rather than fight it. After all, if we can learn to love the difficulties we will inevitably face, then life becomes that much easier, and that much sweeter.

THE PAYOFF

When we are in autopilot mode we have a natural tendency to be negative. Our survival instincts are prone to interpret everyday occurrences as potential dangers and therefore we react to them in an animalistic way.

This is one of the biggest drawbacks of autopilot as it makes us see things as black and white instead of rainbows, and therefore deprives us of a great deal of joy.

Just by noticing when we have a negative reaction and taking a deep breath and smiling, we can escape its clutches more often. By becoming conscious of our internal processing and overcoming its hair-trigger, we will find it so much easier to bounce back from negative experiences, respond and not react and therefore wake up for so much more of our day.

WHAT AM I THINKING?

GIGGLES
AND GUFFAWS

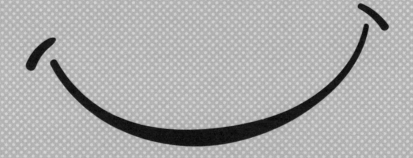

THE INSIGHT

Laughter is said to be the best medicine. Some people seem to do it all the time while others give the impression that their face could never crack a smile without them turning to dust.

Those who laugh more deal with stress better, are healthier and attract more people into their lives. When we share a giggle we connect in a way that is quite unique; something that is deep and true and yet hugely celebratory.

Humour bridges a divide like nothing else. It is not selective by class or race, by gender or age, by profession or stereotype. There is a real human need to have a chuckle, and when we do so, it unites us and makes everything feel OK.

THE PLAN

SHARE A GIGGLE TODAY.

You might tell a joke. You might share a story that somehow tickles folk and helps them smile. You can do anything at all that gets some laughter and spreads a little lightness around your world.

If you're stuck, the internet is packed full of gigglesome things. Don't just watch them on your own, it is important to share the laughs with somebody else. If you really want to push this, then write yourself a little routine and have a go at an open mic night. There really is nothing quite like a few minutes on stage to test your material, and when it goes well little else feels so sweet. If that all feels too much, then just head to a comedy club with a friend and share a joke that way.

THE PAYOFF

Andre Agassi's coach once told him that in life there are two kinds of people: there are thermometers, who can read a room, and then there are thermostats, who can change it. Being able to change the atmosphere is a beautiful gift to have and humour is one of the most fantastic lightning rods of change.

Most of us suffer from taking life too seriously because it's part of the human condition when we are on autopilot. When we laugh, we pop out of that state and wake up while also connecting with ourselves and those people laughing with us.

The more we laugh, the longer we live, and the better every minute feels.

PLUG IN

_____

_____

_____

_____

_____

_____

_____

_____

Smile

THE INSIGHT

When we are taking life too seriously and we feel burdened and heavy we often show it on our faces.

When we smile, however, we get lots of benefits for no effort and no money. Smiling reduces stress and improves your mood; it makes you more creative, more approachable and trustworthy, and improves physiology on a cellular level. In fact, if you smile readily enough you can rewire your brain to become more positive every day, so smiling isn't just for the moment, but for a better life altogether.

So much of our time is spent being transactional and feeling as if we are on our own; yet we know that meaningful human connection has a huge impact on happiness and overall wellbeing. Research has shown that a smile can give people more pleasure than sex, shopping or eating chocolate. In fact, one smile can apparently give people the same amount of stimulation as they would have had from eating 2,000 bars of chocolate, or receiving £16,000 in cash. (How on earth do they measure this stuff?)

Not bad for just cracking a smile.

THE PLAN

SMILE MORE TODAY.

It's important to start this exercise with a little playful cheek. Smiling most certainly will benefit you, but part of the joy is infecting others with it too. Today, make a pact with yourself to try to make everybody you meet smile. If you do this with a friend you can get competitive on how much you touch others, and you may find you learn from their unique techniques and talents. To help remind you not to slip into old ways, draw a smile on one of your hands so that when you see it you are reminded to beam at all those around you with great eye contact and generosity.

THE PAYOFF

Smiling not only makes you feel better by releasing endorphins and reducing cortisol, but also makes other people much warmer towards you and inclined to connect more deeply. You'll feel good, they'll feel good, the world will be a brighter place. And you'll make some new friends.

It's simple but it works.

THE INSIGHT

We all have things we're not proud of in our past.

Nobody leads such a perfect life that everything they do creates unicorns and sunflowers; at times our actions cannot help but deliver gremlins and things that go bump in the night. It is perfectly natural when we look back to wince slightly at our past behaviour and wish that maybe we had played our hand differently.

Regret is something that eats away at us, an energy that is heavy and repressive, and yet it is so easy to shed.

THE PLAN

Think about a moment in your life when you regret how you behaved, a time when, for whatever reason, you did something that doesn't sit right with you today.

As you breathe, smile and remember the details. The recollection may make you uncomfortable but if you hold it, it will eventually settle down as you start to see it for what it was: a mistake and nothing more. Try to connect to the memory of that moment and to who it was that you feel you wronged. As you do so, open your heart and send them unconditional love. If you apologize now energetically, you will feel a large burden lifting.

Now imagine having a conversation with them to put things right between you, so that the regret no longer burns. Depending on who you are and your relationship with that person you have wronged, you may well feel driven to pick up the phone now and set things straight for real. If you do so, bravo! Well done for bringing reconciliation to play. It takes bravery to admit you were wrong and yet pays back in good vibes by the bucketload.

THE PAYOFF

So often we carry unnecessary energy around with us because a little hardship today seems better than facing up to something that seems more painful in the past. You cannot predict how people react to such acts of courage; however, what you can guarantee is that if you do so with good intention the weight will be lifted from your shoulders.

Clearing up your past misdemeanours will help you live life more fully today. Even if you only do it in your imagination and not face-to-face, you can find quiet liberation.

DO
SOMETHING
BIG

THE INSIGHT

When I ask people who have led extraordinary lives what they have done to create such enjoyable experiences, they often reference big changes they have made to their lives.

They may have moved abroad, started a business, learned an unusual skill, followed a passion, thrown it all in and started again. Regardless of the detail, they've all done something large that had risk attached. Interestingly, they often didn't perceive what they were doing as risky but all their friends did. When you ask them why they made that big move the response is usually that it just felt right and it was so damned exciting, they just had to jump. Those decisions are the ones that jolted them out of autopilot into a more profound way of living and helped them to remember that anything is possible.

THE PLAN

Ponder what you might do that would be an absolute game changer for your life. My biggest ones have been getting married, having kids, moving to the seaside, writing my first book, and creating Upping Your Elvis. A good friend of mine has recently taken his kids out of school and gone to Chamonix for the ski season. He tells me it's the biggest boost to his family life, as well as to his work, as he is now invigorated, fresh and full of new thinking for life. He is also no worse off, since the income from renting out his home covered the cost of his accommodation abroad.

What would your big thing be? What could you do that fills you with excitement, because it shows you are truly living your life and not just fitting in with a system that encourages the insidious and gradual creep of autopilot? What is it that can help you remember that you are extraordinary and everything is possible?

Jot down those things that come to mind that are scary, exciting, and yet somehow won't stop calling to you.

Now, what's stopping you? Jump.

THE PAYOFF

We don't always feel ready to do the big stuff, but lack of preparation is often just used as an excuse. The time is never perfect and we can never be absolutely prepared.

Although all the experiments in *Wake Up!* are designed to help counter the dreamlike state we find ourselves in most days, if you really want to jolt your system, do something big.

I threw my job in when I was twenty-seven and went travelling. It was amazing because everything was vibrant, exciting and new. I will always know that it's very easy for me to pack a bag and head off. That option is always within my grasp, so it was worthwhile taking the plunge.

Once you have set up one business, you can set up another. Once you have lived abroad, the whole planet is a possibility. Once you have picked up a new skill, how you spend your time is limitless.

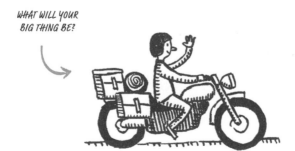

WHAT WILL YOUR
BIG THING BE?

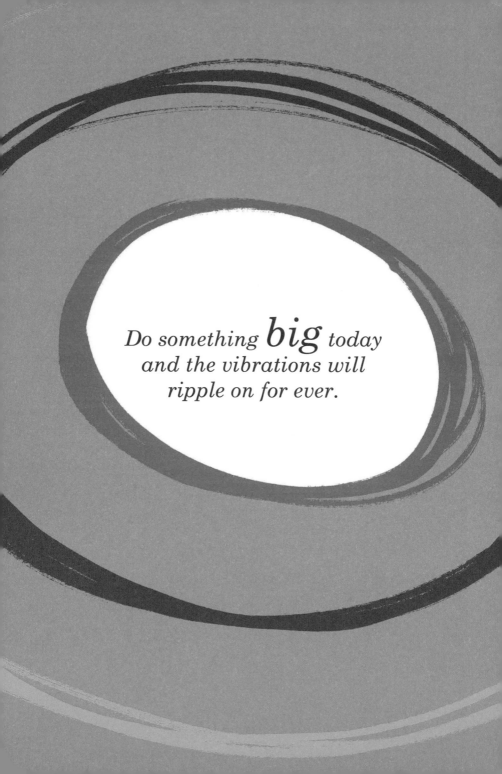

*Do something **big** today and the vibrations will ripple on for ever.*

GUERRILLA

PLANTING

THE INSIGHT

Hell, we can be boring. Subconsciously, there is a crushing pressure upon us to fit in and play nicely. The upside is we live in a polite society, where at least on the surface we all seem civil, but the price is that we forget how fun this life should be.

I am a massive fan of creating a little mischief, especially when that mischief can bring a smile to the faces of others. Guerrilla gardening has been catching people's imaginations and inspiring much spadework for decades. It involves provoking change by bringing nature to spaces where it doesn't exist, such as an inner-city abandoned plot. This isn't an altogether modern phenomenon; its history stretches back as far as a rebel horticulturalist known as the Digger in Surrey in 1649. The key is that you don't have permission to plant and yet whatever grows adds natural beauty to that space.

Of course, I am not condoning vandalism or destruction. Guerrilla gardening should always be carried out responsibly, using plants that are suitable for the site with the aim of making an improvement rather than creating a problem.

THE PLAN

THIS WEEK WE WILL ALL BECOME GUERRILLA GARDENERS IN OUR OWN LITTLE WAY.

We don't need to create masterpieces like the famous Adam Purple's Garden of Eden, which ended up covering over 15,000 square feet in Manhattan; we just need to plant something, somewhere surprising.

We can all find an empty space that needs some colour. Be creative; many pavements have patches of soil around unloved trees just shouting out for a shot of green finery. I like the idea of planting seeds or bulbs that take a while to flourish, as the anticipation of knowing they will burst into bloom at some later unspecified date is as much a joy as when they finally do, but I know that for many planters there is huge fun in putting something more substantial in the ground.

THE PAYOFF

When we feel slightly nervous and excited we often
feel a little more alive, and while our guerrilla
planting shouldn't really upset anyone, it is for
sure a little bit naughty. Doing something fun and
frivolous can remind us that this life is supposed to
be a party and not something that should be hard,
arduous and troublesome.

I also get a kick out of someone else noticing a splash
of beauty in a place where, strictly, it shouldn't be.
Maybe, it will help them wake up too.

Stay Still
AND SOAK IT UP

THE INSIGHT

When we rush around we become part of the chaotic soup of existence. It's impossible to appreciate that soup when you are swimming in it. If, however, you step back and observe its motion, the perspective helps you remember how its ingredients combine.

We have numerous levels of awareness. Much of our lives are spent feeling as if we are on our own – and indeed, we are purely the person we see in the mirror every day. When we are swept up in that soup, it reinforces the view that life should be difficult, fast and tricky. Equally, most of us are fully aware that there is more to us than just our physical bodies, the jobs we do and the lives we lead, and that we are connected to something much bigger. Stepping out of the soup can help us remember that.

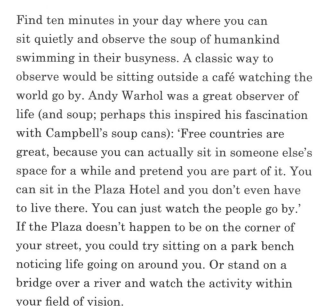

THE PLAN

Find ten minutes in your day where you can sit quietly and observe the soup of humankind swimming in their busyness. A classic way to observe would be sitting outside a café watching the world go by. Andy Warhol was a great observer of life (and soup; perhaps this inspired his fascination with Campbell's soup cans): 'Free countries are great, because you can actually sit in someone else's space for a while and pretend you are part of it. You can sit in the Plaza Hotel and you don't even have to live there. You can just watch the people go by.' If the Plaza doesn't happen to be on the corner of your street, you could try sitting on a park bench noticing life going on around you. Or stand on a bridge over a river and watch the activity within your field of vision.

Do not distract yourself with conversation or those little electronic devices; just soak it all up and notice how when you sit quietly and breathe well (see Learn to Breathe! on page 28) you are in a very different energetic state from the rest of the world that is flowing past you.

THE PAYOFF

A few moments in your day stepping back from the commotion is a brilliant anchor in obtaining consciousness and choice. It may seem like an opulent indulgence, but for me it's the equivalent of meditation. Often people feel as if to calm the mind, they have to go inside, but with this simple activity you'll find that the busyness of the outside can produce the inner calm you desire. Neat and easy and effective.

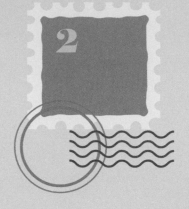

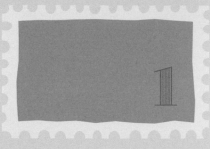

WRITE A
LETTER
TO SOMEONE
YOU CARE ABOUT

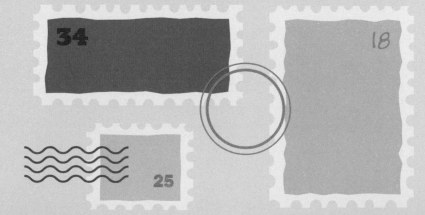

THE INSIGHT

The human race is becoming ever more independent and isolated. The number of us living on our own continues to increase and social interaction is plummeting owing to the increased physical separation of the digital age.

When Sir Tim Berners Lee invented the World Wide Web, its mission was to serve humanity and to connect not just machines, but people. The internet, used wisely, does this and more. Like anything, when we overuse it, we create a problem for ourselves. Analogue mediums help ground us and reconnect us with our natural human instincts.

We aren't spending enough time with the people who count, and that often means we're not talking about what's important. Amy Winehouse had 10 million likes on her Facebook, yet she died alone, watching YouTube videos of herself. That can't be right. To be happy, fulfilled and properly connected to this planet we need to have meaningful relationships in our lives.

THE PLAN

THIS WEEK WRITE A LETTER TO SOMEBODY THAT YOU CARE ABOUT. THE LETTER CAN BE ABOUT ANYTHING AT ALL, AS LONG AS IT INCLUDES ONE THING YOU TRULY APPRECIATE ABOUT THE PERSON YOU'RE WRITING TO.

Take your time. Letters are written so rarely now, it is right to luxuriate in the experience and make each word count. When we write a letter, we slow down time. We first have to value that communication and to clear some space to do it. Physically writing a letter means that we connect more with what we are saying and then, as we lick the envelope, seal it and take it to the post box, there is an exquisite and necessary delay in gratification. These windows of time are luxurious and worth rolling around in.

WHO WOULD YOU WRITE
YOUR LETTER TO?

THE PAYOFF

By taking the time to write to somebody you care about, you start to appreciate more of what it is that makes them special and what it is they give to you. By appreciating that, you will feel more connected to them and will be more grateful. They will also enjoy the wonderful benefits of being cared for and acknowledged, and it will help them be more awake when they read it. When you read a letter like that, the day is instantly more colourful.

The Tagalog word for 'unhappy' is the same as 'lonely', but you don't have to come from the Philippines to understand why. Real connections count; it's what life is about.

My grandfather only ever wrote me one letter. I still have it.

WHY NOW?

The game of life used to be all about achievement. To win we had to follow the rules and a rather linear path to success.

Obviously, we needed to flourish in school, and we knew that a well-rounded education created a well-rounded individual. Flourishing unique talents and left-field passions were suppressed in order that we would all fit in nicely and learn how to regurgitate facts beautifully with little understanding of why they might be useful. We had to eradicate our weaknesses and then, as an all-rounder, we could proceed through the multi-level educational system and be deposited on the other side ready to join the world's workforce.

Under that system, careers were all about progression. Your first job generally sucked, and the rest of your working life was spent trying to get a job that sucked a little less and paid a little more. We were conditioned to aspire to a life path of marriage, mortgage, parenthood and holidays abroad while keeping up with the Joneses. Once we'd achieved that, our next project would be, of course, to ensure that our children were raised to become well-rounded future members of the world's workforce . . .

The board game of life was laid out before us. We all knew the rules and every year we'd roll the dice and see how far we'd move. Because we knew where we were going, we didn't have to think too much, or indeed be aware of alternative paths.

But that was then, and this is now. The days of the linear life are ending. Our education system is failing and our children can often learn more from YouTube than from their teachers.

A life where you have only one job with a set salary is no longer the norm for many. There is an awareness that achieving more, earning more, owning more and consuming more will only take us into oblivion. We have to start living every day well if we are to honour the precious life that we are the guardians of. Escaping autopilot means that we can truly be who we are and challenge the norms from which we can now all break free.

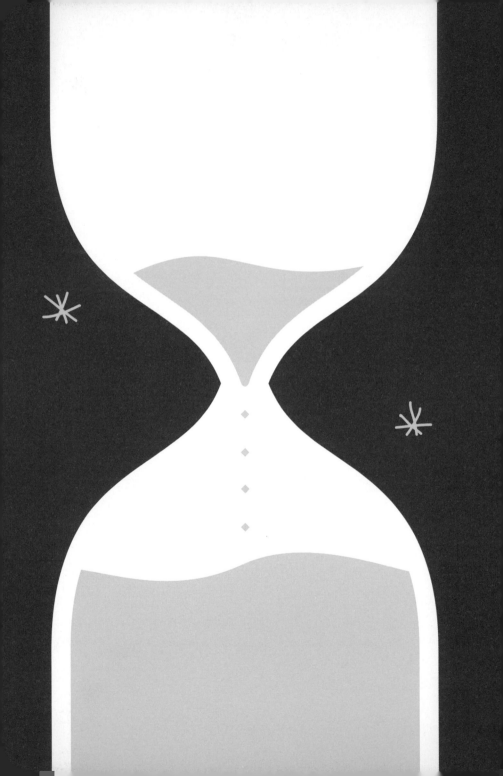

Time is limited.
Let's not waste it.

AND
SOON
WE WILL DIE

THE INSIGHT

I once read that life is short and life is long, but not in that order. It does resonate with me, as when I was younger I felt that my lifetime was almost infinite as it stretched into the future. I was invincible and everything was a possibility. I felt there was no rush or panic to use my time well as I possessed it in abundance, and therefore a day on the sofa recovering from excesses seemed nothing more than a little pit stop.

Nowadays, my responsibilities have grown and my time has become more pressured, so it would seem the years pass faster; so fast that it can seem as if life is purely about busyness rather than truly living. Autopilot loves it when we have too much on because we have no choice but to engage in it, just to cope with our day-to-day activity.

When we consider that we don't have that many days on this planet (29,565 on average in the UK, and around a third of those are spent at work), it can help us remember that each day is precious and that each one has to count.

THE PLAN

SIT QUIETLY SOMEWHERE YOU HAVE A VIEW OF THE EARTH AND THE SKY, TAKE A DEEP BREATH AND THEN PONDER THAT YOUR DEATH IS INEVITABLE.

It may not be for a hundred years with the amazing advances of technology, but equally it could be in a hundred days or a hundred seconds, because that's the way the dice roll.

With that in mind, what should you be doing today that would make it a great day?

It may not be an action or an activity or a thing that you need to achieve; it may very well be how you are and what you appreciate. We only have so many conversations with our loved ones, how can today's count? We only drink so many cups of tea, how can we really enjoy this one? We only take so many walks, why is today's special?

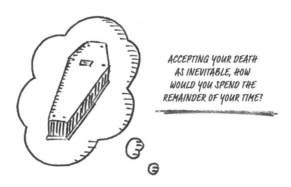

ACCEPTING YOUR DEATH
AS INEVITABLE, HOW
WOULD YOU SPEND THE
REMAINDER OF YOUR TIME?

THE PAYOFF

David Bowie was one of my heroes. He died at sixty-nine. Did someone you know or admire die young? It may not happen to you, but it could. If I were to mirror Bowie, that would give me only another twenty-one years. That probably means another ten years of working full on; and that probably means I will write only three more books. That kind of thinking is a real eye-opener. It makes me realize I should probably be dicking around a hell of a lot more and loving every second . . . and it certainly means I should be spending more time with my family, properly connected and rolling around in the joy of it. Useful perspective.

I was recently asked about my ambition and I realized that it was no longer about achieving more, becoming better and all that striving for greatness, but it was about living well today. By remembering that we are not here for an infinite number of days, maybe we can all do that bit better by spending those we do have more awake.

WAKEY WAKEY

Every day on this planet should be extraordinary. Not in a 'tickertape parade, high-fiving whoop-de-doo' type way, but in an 'enjoying being alive for what it is' kind of way.

Each one of these exercises has been fun for me and in writing this book and trying them out I've discovered that the exercises in themselves were not the lesson. Rather, by trying these different things, and having a right good laugh in doing so, I have remembered what it is about life that I love so much. We have unlimited opportunities for fun. We have unlimited opportunities to meet amazing people. We have unlimited opportunities to feel truly awake every single day, and I believe that when you value that and you have connected to that belief sufficiently deeply, you will never let a day go by without tasting it.

I am now committed to keep experimenting for the rest of my days, and I hope that you will come along on the journey with me. My dream is that like-minded people will share their experiments with us all, so that together we can try new and different ways of waking up. There are absolutely no rules to how this works. Readers have bent, broken and reinvented these exercises hundreds of times already and each incarnation brings a unique benefit.

When we get creative and help others tap into that genius, we can only get better at breaking away from autopilot and learning more deeply, so I hope you will be part of the community that takes on that mantle and keeps alive what I have started.

Please join us here and try out other people's tips and share your learnings too, if you fancy.

There is nothing sacred about this book beyond its attitude. I believe that we all have the opportunity to be amazing and to lead lives of legend. If we embrace the energy of what is written in this book, we have a much greater chance to have a grin on our face and a skip in our step.

If enough of us do this every day and truly wake up, this world will not spin just a little bit better but it will start to right its wrongs and value life the way it should be valued. If you want to plug in to the extraordinary and the Technicolor and don't want to waste another minute of this most amazing time that we are here on this planet, *Wake Up!*

ACKNOWLEDGEMENTS

I am very proud of this book but I can't take credit for it.

I am blessed to laugh more often than is sanctioned and I am blessed to have such amazing people in my life who have loved, supported, stimulated, inspired, put back on track, prodded and poked me to where I am today and have made this book happen.

I am truly grateful for all your genius.

Huge thanks to those who have made a very direct input to *Wake Up!*, both the book and the platform. I always miss some out, please forgive me, but they include Gemma Greaves, Michael Acton-Smith, Colin Corbridge, Josh and all at Crowdhub, Dan Keiran, Shilen Patel, Gordon Peterson, Chris Goldson, Steve Gladdis, David Micklem, David Pappa, Andy Bradley, David Pearl and all at Street Wisdom, Fi McWilliam, Emma Snellgrove, Mel McDougall, Nicca Kathrens, Dr Mark Fowlestone, Prof. Paul Dolan, Kris Murrin, David McCready, Guy Escolme, Scott Hunter and Monty and Ian and team, Andy Reid, Mike DaRe, Joel Rickett and Emily Robertson from Penguin, Trevor Horwood and my rather exceptional brother, Mark.

Big thanks to Purdeys, Finisterre, Quoddy's, Hiut Denim, John Vavatros, Blok Knives and Tesla for making lovely things and helping me out!

The award for most ridiculous contribution goes to Vanessa Barlow, who not only researched, edited and promoted it, but kept me honest and true. No mean feat.

To Suzy Greaves and all at *Psychologies* magazine for letting me experiment with you and importantly to the bloggers and readers who have done these experiments and have helped make them better. Thanks for having the faith.

To all of those who have trusted me enough to keep me doing my work. There are lots of you but a special thanks to Karen Blackett, Kelly Williams and Simon Daglish, Stan Sthanunathan, Christina Habib and Jen Whyte, Matt Barwell, Clare Owen, Charlie Downing, Maria Eitel, the ever mighty Keith Wilmot and so many more who are ripping up the rule book and making work a more human and fun place to be.

To all at Upping Your Elvis. Without Matt, Harriet and Alex it couldn't be done. And thanks to Jim who is bullet proof, larger than life and lives Elvis every day. A great friend, and a proper gent.

And, of course, to my family. My folks have been amazing; I can't thank you enough for the unconditional love and support even in the face of my constant lunacy.

To Louli, who makes my heart leap whenever I see her and taught me about that unconditional love that my folks do so well. Harvey, who has shown me what creativity really is and that being true to yourself is what we need to deliver every single day if we are to shine.

To Anna, my gorgeous wife. Words ain't enough. I am so smitten and so grateful. Thank you for showing me the way and for making me bigger . . .

And lastly, thanks to you.

Without you having the drive and desire to challenge what is usually accepted and to work out your own truth, *Wake Up!* would be for nothing.

Keep shining bright and loving every minute of it.

But now it's your turn.

I WOULD LIKE TO THANK MYSELF BECAUSE . . .

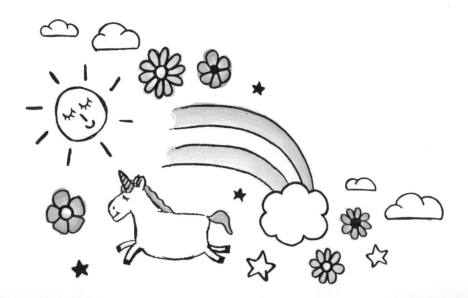